THE UNCERTAIN ART

THE
UNCERTAIN ART

THOUGHTS ON A LIFE IN MEDICINE

Sherwin B. Nuland

RANDOM HOUSE NEW YORK

Published in the United States by Random House,
an imprint of The Random House Publishing Group, a division of
Random House, Inc., New York.

RANDOM HOUSE and colophon are registered trademarks of
Random House, Inc.

All the pieces in this work, with the exception of "Letters from a
Heart Transplant Candidate," which appears for the first time here,
were originally published in *The American Scholar.*

ISBN 978-1-4000-6478-6

Printed in the United States of America on acid-free paper

www.atrandom.com

2 4 6 8 9 7 5 3 1

FIRST EDITION

Book design by Simon M. Sullivan

To those "who taught me this Art."

—FROM THE HIPPOCRATIC OATH

CONTENTS

Author's Note	xi
Prooemium: An Introduction to My Book	xiii
THE WHOLE LAW OF MEDICINE	3
NARCISSUS LOOKS INTO THE LABORATORY	12
THE MEDICAL SCHOOL AND THE UNIVERSITY	20
THE TRUE HEALERS	28
PUMPING IRON	35
ACUPUNCTURE IN THE OPERATING ROOM	42
CHINESE MEDICINE, WESTERN SCIENCE, AND ACUPUNCTURE	50
THE MISTY CRYSTAL BALL	59
HIDDEN MEANINGS	67
IS THERE A DOCTOR IN THE HOUSE?	75
WRITING	83
ROBBING GRAVES	91
MIND, BODY, AND THE DOCTOR	99
THE GREAT BOOKS	108
GRIEF AND REFLECTION: AFTER 9/11	116
LIGHTNING ON MY MIND	123

Scatological Medicine   132

Hippocrates Redux   140

The Artist and the Doctor   148

The Man or the Moment?   157

Letters from a Heart Transplant Candidate   165

Acknowledgments   187

Index   189

AUTHOR'S NOTE

This book consists almost entirely of a series of essays as they appeared in *The American Scholar* between 1998 and 2004. As I read through them today, I realize that some of the hopes expressed here are already in the early stages of being fulfilled, while others are as far from fruition as they were when first proposed. They represent the Art, as Hippocrates called medicine, seen by an ardent admirer and unsparing critic—a man honored to have participated in its daily wonders and uncertainties for half a century. They tell of the practice of medicine as I have observed it and loved it—and lived it.

The final story has not previously been published. It is written in tribute to a brave man who became my friend during the final period of his life, a man I respected as I have few others. When certain of the expectations appearing in this book reach a state of practical usefulness, the day will come when no man, woman, or child will die awaiting the transplantation of a donor organ. May that day be soon.

PROOEMIUM

AN INTRODUCTION TO MY BOOK

There is wisdom in the acceptance of uncertainty. Well used, it can make a philosopher of an ordinary man. To the intuitive mind of the twenty-two-year-old John Keats, that precious insight appeared in a flash of understanding one day in 1817, while he was deep in conversation on a long walk with two friends: "[S]everal things dove-tailed in my mind, and at once it struck me what quality went to form a man of achievement," he later wrote in a letter to his brothers. "I mean *negative capability*, that is, when a man is capable of being in uncertainties, mysteries, doubts." To become comfortable with uncertainty is one of the primary goals in the training of a physician.

Keats wrote those words—italics and all—during the period when he was composing *Endymion*. Less than a year earlier, he had stopped attending the series of lectures that were to prepare him for the examinations of the Royal College of Surgeons. Although poetry and the pursuit of sunbeams had long since become Keats's passions, he had been anything but an indifferent student. The statements of contemporaries attest to his skillful performance of clinical duties, and he had already qualified to practice medicine in July 1816, following a year's study at Guy's Hospital. Medical education was brief in those days. Although the examinations were difficult, there was little of real usefulness to learn.

It was not possible for a perceptive man to study medicine in the early nineteenth century without becoming aware of the degree to which patient care was conducted in a pervasive atmosphere of inexactness. Like all young doctors of the time, Keats very likely admired his teachers at Guy's all the more for their ability not only to be decisive in the face of uncertainty but actually to thrive in the absence of clear clinical signposts. Even the basic principles of physical examination were not well known by most doctors, this being the period when they were originally introduced—and in Paris, no less. It was in 1816, in fact, that René Laënnec, a Breton who at five feet three inches was almost as diminutive as Keats himself, invented the stethoscope.

For physicians, the nineteenth century was characterized by the gradual infiltration of new scientific findings into medical thought. The process accelerated rapidly in the 1880s and 1890s, as the products of laboratory investigations in physiology and bacteriology were finally shown to be of practical use at the bedside. By the first decade of the twentieth century, an increasingly credible, scientifically based medicine had routed the forces of homeopathy and the other irregular sects that, until then, had retained some hope of gaining ascendancy. From that point onward, the Holy Grail would be a form of practice based on knowledge gained by observation, hypothesis, experiment, and verification, in which uncertainty, if a factor at all, would be quickly dispersed by the next series of laboratory or epidemiological studies—a discipline, in other words, that might with real justification be called a science.

Yet even with an expanding population of trained researchers and increased funding for medical education and research, wise observers recognized the existence of problems unique to the practice of medicine that would forever frustrate its hopes of becoming a true science. Dr. William Osler of Johns Hopkins, at the time the most scientifically advanced American medical school, pointed this out on several occasions. "[W]ho can tell of the uncertainties of medicine as an art?" he asked rhetorically of an audience of physicians in 1903. "The science on which it is based is accurate and definite enough . . . [but] no two individuals react alike and behave alike under the abnormal conditions which we know as disease." He spoke that day of "this everlasting *perhaps* with which we have to preface so much connected with the practice of our art." Osler lauded the pursuit of probability, recognizing that to pursue certainty is to chase after an illusion. In this, he was no more than echoing the First Aphorism of Hippocrates, written 2,400 years earlier: "Life is short, and the Art is long; the occasion fleeting; experience fallacious, and judgment difficult."

It is judgment that lies at the heart of diagnosis, of therapy, and of all that is gathered under the umbrella of what clinicians call case management. Inherent in the nature of clinical decision making is the realization that, perforce, it must always be accomplished in the face of incomplete and largely ambiguous information. The process is one of sifting, weighing, and judging and will ever be thus. Disease never reveals all of itself; the path toward healing may appear visible, but it is always poorly lit and subject to changes in direction. No matter what biomedical advances may realistically be expected in the future, no one who has spent more than a few months at the bedsides of the sick could find it conceivable that this imperfect state of affairs will ever change. Uncertainty is more than a constant—it is the very muse that inspires the intellectual fascination of medical practice. To accept it is the essence of wisdom; to *enjoy* it is the essence of the enrichment of a doctor's soul, exceeded only by the personal reward of helping a fellow human being in trouble. Without uncertainty there would be no need for judgment; without judgment, medicine would be a career for technicians, and, given the intrinsic nature of illness, an impossibility.

More than a hundred years have passed since Osler spoke of the uncertainty inherent in the art of medicine. Surely, one might ask, has not the exponential increase in scientific knowledge in the intervening time, especially during the past five decades, vastly changed the situation? Do we not nowadays have access to sources of information that have markedly decreased the uncertainty? The answer to both questions, of course, is yes. But the operative words are "changed" and "decreased"— not "erased." For as long as there is individual variability in human biology; in the specific manifestations of any given disease; in the social setting in which the disease occurs; in the psychological response to disease; and, in turn, the feedback effect of that response on the disease and the patient's perception of it—as long as all those differentiating and problematic factors exist, as they will forever, there can be no certainty in medicine, and medicine will remain an art rather than a science.

But what of the allegedly undisputable nature of the evidence on which so much of so-called scientific medicine is based? On close inspection, much of that turns out to be disputable and even undependable. In a word, uncertain. Were it not, medical theory would not be subject to the frequent oscillations in diagnostic and therapeutic thinking that have characterized it in our era. In recent decades, for example, we have witnessed wide swings of expert opinion on such matters as the proper treatment of breast cancer, the cause of peptic ulcer, and the future of infectious diseases, about all of which physicians had previously felt quite certain. Other sacred cows will no doubt stop producing milk in the coming years. The single certainty is uncertainty. Only the reliability of unreliability is to be relied on.

Medical interventions and instrumentation have traditionally entered the canon of usage without fulfilling criteria that would satisfy even the least demanding of bench scientists. Satisfaction with immediate and early results, absence of obvious harm, and habits of long custom have sufficed to keep therapies in the current arsenal and discouraged critical questioning of their efficacy. As surprising as it may be to the general public and even to many physicians, medical methods and theory stand on far less firm ground than is generally realized. Although science is the most highly regarded ingredient (with personal experience a powerful second), large if unrecognized dollops of individual bias, authoritarianism, cultural values, and even emotion find their way into bedside lucubrations. Every one of these factors—including those that on the surface seem unqualifiedly negative—has its own benefits. Each, including science and experience, likewise brings its own innate problems into the mix. When one or several ingredients inevitably change with the passage of time, medical fashions change with them. As Lynn C. Epstein, associate dean of medicine at Brown University, has so aptly put it, "While the continuing gains in medical knowledge and the accompanying ability of doctors to treat the sick have been real, the passage of time has too often proven the espoused remedies of one era to be of limited value or frankly harmful in the next. . . . How much of what we embrace as truth today will suffer this fate over the ensuing decades?"

Geography counts too. Significant variations in methods of treating the same disease have been shown to occur in different cities, indicating that what might be called the local medical culture is a real factor in the choices physicians make. The glaring spotlight of official attention has now been turned on such issues of medical uncertainty. Recognizing how few clinical interventions are supported by valid evidence of their long-term usefulness, the federal government established the Agency for Healthcare Research and Quality, to study the late effects of various medical methods. The field of so-called outcomes research—in which large numbers of patients are studied over extended periods of time in an attempt to find out what really happens when one or another treatment is used—is now all the rage.

And even after such investigations have been conducted for decades, to what use can the agency's critical evaluations be put in the case of any specific patient? Though the advent of correctives such as the randomized controlled clinical trial and the newly popular notion of evidence-based medicine may have lessened the uncertainty inherent in general principles of therapy, they are unlikely—for the reasons given in preceding paragraphs—to usefully affect the care of an individual man, woman, or child to the degree claimed or predicted by their most adamant advocates. Given the spectrum of illness presentations, we will be left with what we have always had and always will have—the acceptance of the long-established principle that the practice of medicine is characterized by uncertainty and will always require judgment in order to be effective. That is its very nature.

Not only is the management of disease itself uncertain, but even the proper domain of medical responsibility is hazily demarcated and subject to vigorous debate. Every decade finds the boundaries extended of what is thought to correctly fall within the realm of a doctor's concerns. Today, it is no longer enough to diagnose and treat organic and mental pathologies. Doctors are involved in a wide variety of problems that in previous eras were left to be solved personally or by families, social agencies or government bureaus. An organization of physicians, International Physicians for the Prevention of Nuclear War, has even won the Nobel Peace Prize for its ban-the-bomb activities, in 1985.

Whether or not one feels these subjects are appropriate for white-coated attention, the fact is that ours is an increasingly medicalized society.

Even our notions of what constitutes an illness are widening. Who in Osler's day would have consulted a doctor because he was unhappy about the shape of his nose or unable to achieve a satisfactory erection at the age of sixty? Some of the change is the result of new technology, but some is symptomatic of the temper of our time, in which anything that causes human unhappiness is unacceptable, and therefore a fair target for the physician. And some of the change is based simply on what insurance companies will pay for. Before the general advent of third-party payers, no one took a child to the emergency room because of a scraped knee.

Clearly, the definitions of medicine's limits are uncertain nowadays. So vaguely defined have they become that the Hastings Institute, America's premier bioethics think tank, some years ago conducted an international effort called the Project on the Goals of Medicine, seeking to arrive at answers to such basic questions as just what it is that medicine should be trying to do for individuals and for the greater society. Not surprisingly, the results have been indecisive and even uncertain. To the average physician of today, the boundaries of professional responsibility and jurisdiction are anything but clear.

All of this is a prologue to introducing the substance of my book and explaining the title I have chosen for it. By now it is doubtless clear that *The Uncertain Art* refers to medicine and that I have been attempting in the foregoing paragraphs to stake out a territory whose boundaries are sufficiently vague that I may feel free to roam wherever inclination leads me. Roam, that is, so long as I stay within sight of the assignment I have given myself, which is to write as a doctor, about issues associated with doctoring.

I have chosen to interpret that word—"doctoring"—in its broadest sense, the sense of the entire spectrum of what should concern the doctor whom any of us might ideally seek out to be the caretaker of our own health. By this, I mean a man or woman trained as a physician but committed as much to the humanism of medicine as to the science. And as for science itself, I interpret that heading to include both the microcosm and the macrocosm. So many far-flung aspects of scientific study influence biomedicine and clinical practice nowadays that none of its branches can be excluded. Our Hippocratic forebears and our colleagues who use non-Western forms of treatment have made much of the interrelationships between the health of individuals and humankind's participation in nature's surrounding universe, and I intend to do no less. Moreover, Keats having been invoked in this very first chapter, I have set a precedent for straying untethered when the impulse strikes, as have so many of the literary doctors of the past. In this, I turn for validation to such as William Carlos Williams, MD, who said of his daily medical round, "[I]t was my very food and drink, the very thing which made it possible for me to write." The art of medicine is a crucible, into which go and out of which come the mixtures that make life.

Just as medicine has permeated every aspect of our society, so the process of extending outward the free association of a doctor's concerns will allow for much that might seem far afield. During the first century c.e., the Roman scholar Celsus produced a three-volume work intended to describe for the general reader all that was then known of the art of healing. He was not a physician but a member of that small band whom students of the classical period call encyclopedists; his *De medicina* is encyclopedic. It deals with every aspect of sickness, health, medical history, philosophy, and ethics in which an ordinary citizen might be interested. When I began planning this book, I could not help remembering Celsus. Though his work is not exactly a prototype for what I hope to accomplish here, his breadth of vision about what constitutes the arena of medical concerns provides a framework for my subject's ramifications, or at least a background against which to consider them. It was in recalling Celsus that I chose to entitle this first chapter "Prooemium," as he called the preface in which he outlined his notions of the scope of medicine and his intentions for the writings. In my own "Prooemium," I have tried to do just that.

Celsus stayed within the admittedly wide boundaries he set for himself, and it is my intention to do the same. Yet it may be that this book will one day be thought to have needed its own Project on Goals, should I at some future time be found to have strayed willy-nilly beyond the fuzzy edges of even the most extensive of frontiers. But when I consider the vastness of the constantly increasing territory that I can legitimately claim as my own—and the generosity with which the fruitful landscape has been endowed—that day would seem to be far off, if indeed it ever comes.

THE UNCERTAIN ART

THE WHOLE LAW OF MEDICINE

Life is short, and the Art is long; the occasion fleeting; experience falla-
cious, and judgment difficult. The physician must not only be prepared
to do what is right himself, but also to make the patient, the attendants,
and the externals, cooperate.

THE FIRST APHORISM
ATTRIBUTED TO HIPPOCRATES, C. 400 B.C.E.

It has long been accepted that a considerable portion of the body of
writings credited to Hippocrates was in fact authored by others, in
the two centuries following his death. But until recent decades, scholars remained convinced that reliable criteria were recognizable by
which at least a certain core of the material might still be identified as
his own. They set this group of texts off from the rest by calling it
"The Genuine Works of Hippocrates."

English translations of these central teachings were inadequate and
incomplete until the mid-nineteenth century, when the Sydenham
Society of London commissioned the Scottish surgeon Francis Adams
to provide a definitive edition. Published in 1849, the two-volume
result of Adams's efforts—naturally called *The Genuine Works of
Hippocrates*—took its place as the authentic historic record.

During the last century, cracks began to appear in the supposed evidence by which some of even these "genuine" works had been certified
into the canon, but the short book of pithy clinical maxims known as
The Aphorisms held out longer than most. As recently as 1934, members of America's first think tank of medical historians, based at Johns
Hopkins University, could write in their *Bulletin:* "It is almost universally agreed that among the many Hippocratic writings, the *Aphorisms*

are genuine." The editors of the journal then went on to point out something that remains true to this day: "They are also undoubtedly by far the most popular books; printed, translated, and commented upon endless times, they were the physician's bible for many centuries." And in a little aside, they added the surprising—at least to me—statement that the introduction into English of the very word "aphorism" is owed to this "anthology of medical truths."

Nowadays, finding a historian who agrees that *The Aphorisms* was actually written by the legendary Father of Medicine is as unlikely as finding a clinical physician who agrees that all of the 422 nuggets of advice contained in its pages are "medical truths." Though enshrined in the tradition of almost two and a half millennia as the First Aphorism of Hippocrates, the words of this chapter's epigraph, for example, were probably never uttered by their putative author. A few reasonably dependable bits of information are known about the great man's life: he was born about 460 B.C.E. on the Greek island of Cos; he was probably an itinerant physician; he seems to have been a leader in the formation of a school for the training of young doctors. We know little more than that, and what we do know most assuredly does not include hard evidence that Hippocrates left any identifiable corpus of written work. As for the clinical pearls of wisdom: although some of them are nothing less than astonishing in the accuracy of their perceptiveness and the wisdom of their recommendations, others are so bewilderingly at odds with simple observation that they seem to have been inserted to keep the reader awake by making him laugh. What, for example, is a doctor to do with such pronouncements as "The bald are not subject to varicose veins" and "Stammerers are particularly liable to obstinate diarrhea"?

All this having been said, the First Aphorism continues to stand by itself as a model of, of—well, of precisely that: the perfect aphorism, well deserving of its priority, which, if that 1934 issue of the *Bulletin of the Institute for the History of Medicine* is to be believed, places it squarely as being indeed *the* first of all time. An aphorism *should* stand by itself, without reference to anything preceding or following it, and it must express a timeless truth in a brief burst of sagacity, requiring no editorializing, interpretation, or further comment.

But of course, the more memorable the aphorism, the more likely it is that editorializing, interpretation, and further comment will be its fate in perpetuity. Particularly when the epigrammatic saying incorporates principles that have guided a profession for two thousand years, as this one has, there is no end to the ways in which it is likely to be studied, discussed, and anatomized. Add to this its source in a classical language spoken by very few of those who would dissect its lesson, and the result is countless pages and perorations that have never added an iota of substance to the original.

In this it resembles the Hippocratic Oath, which has also been the object of much learned discourse and even a good deal of fretting, especially in today's ferment of anxious debate over assisted suicide, abortion, and other ethical issues for which the profession and the public seek a precedent in time-honored codes of behavior, or at least a guide to immutable principles of morality. Ethicists and others have worried the Oath as a dog worries a bone, craving the meat and marrow of some eternal principia with which to strengthen the ancient bonds of professional obligation. Yet even as their elders cleave to the Oath, recent classes of graduating medical students have not hesitated to "bring the text up to date" or "make it relevant to our needs" in order to reflect whatever acceptable current values they are willing to espouse in this self-absorbed era of moral relativism. Like scripture, the Oath is quoted by both sinners and saints. For every traditionalist, there is a revisionist who claims it to be interpretable or amenable to alteration as needed, often in ways different from what its original words would seem to imply. There is even a body of historical opinion holding that in its day, large sections (or perhaps all) of it were ignored by most physicians. But here the case of the First Aphorism differs markedly from that of the Oath: though it has been the subject of plenty of discussion, there is little disagreement over the aphorism's intent.

Clearly, the First Aphorism was written by one or more wise and vastly experienced physicians, but its purpose was not to provide a moral precept. It was meant simply as a statement of what it is like to try to care for the sick. Not only does the aphorism avoid preachiness, but, quite to the contrary, it is a testimony to the humility with which a doctor should approach his calling and a declaration of the profession's delineated capabilities. Its subtext is the very basis upon which this book has been given its title: the uncertainty inherent in the art of medicine.

In my view, the First Aphorism should be read to every beginning class on its initial morning of medical school. A student is then still a "civilian," one who has not yet absorbed so much as a particle of that fluctuating mix of science and art of which the profession has always consisted. From that hour forward, the values of the guild will soak ever more deeply into his or her mind and self-image, so that the end of the first academic year finds a young person vastly transformed. It would be good for that transformation to start with the First Aphorism—at the very least, a dawning of insight into what must be borne in mind if the task ahead is to be accomplished with scientific skill and humanity both, and with tolerance for the Art's limitations as well as one's own. It would be good, too, if the aphorism were to be reread yearly or even more often, that it might fix itself into the perceptions of the developing doctor so steadfastly as to remain ever in the forefront of thought. Like the Talmudic sage Hillel's response when he was challenged to summarize his religion while standing on one foot—that one never do to others what is hateful to oneself—the First Aphorism is medicine's whole law; the rest is commentary. Having learned that law, one should (as Hillel enjoined his challenger after both feet were back on the ground) go and study it.

The thing needs to be parsed. In doing so, I will deliberately avoid certain venerable scholarly differences of opinion about the proper translation of a few of the aphorism's words, relying instead on the English as it appears in the original Adams publication, which, with slight variations, is the commonly accepted version. At first, I will restrict my comments to the statement's first sentence. Life may be short, but I plan to make mine long enough to get back to that vastly important second section in a later chapter.

Life is short, and the Art is long. Although life expectancy is currently well more than twice what it was during the golden age of Greece, it will never be endowed with years enough for anyone to master the vast expanse of medical knowledge, or even that part of it sufficient for an individual doctor to care for all of his patients. In every era, some people live well beyond their expected span; Hippocrates himself seems to have been one hundred when he died in approximately 360 B.C.E. Yet even at the barest beginning of Western medicine's history, it was recognized that no man's lifetime was sufficient to learn all that was required.

In view of what comes next, it is pertinent to point out that some commentators have read these opening words in a different way, taking their meaning to be that medicine demands a certain amount of time to exert its healing powers, but the patient's life may be short once disease strikes. Either way, there is a realization here of the inconsistency between the time required and the time available, a factor over which no physician has control.

The occasion fleeting. Here, too, the focus is the urgency that exists in most medical situations, even those that are not acute emergencies. There is a finite period in the course of a disease (and for some, "fleeting" is indeed appropriate) when it is amenable to curative treatment. Although the window is considerably larger now in the early twenty-first century, it is well known that timely diagnosis is often a greater factor in outcome than is the treatment per se. When a patient presents himself to the physician beyond a certain point in the evolution of a disease process, the opportunity for a satisfactory result is diminished or lost. When statisticians in the Department of Health Studies at the University of Chicago pointed out in *The New England Journal of Medicine* that evaluations of cancer mortality in the United States between 1970 and 1994 demonstrated a "lack of substantial improvement over what treatment could already accomplish some decades ago," they pointed out that the best therapeutic methods and prevention must be accompanied by "access to the earliest possible diagnosis." Looking from the opposite perspective, I have in my own career witnessed a decline in the long-term mortality rate of women with breast cancer, attributable for the most part to the fact that patients began in the late

1970s and early 1980s to be diagnosed at an earlier stage of the disease, thanks to increased public discussion and the widespread introduction of effective mammography.

Preach though he may about the necessity of early discovery and intervention, the physician may find that achieving this goal in an individual case is, by and large, beyond his control if his patient is not alert and informed. Even then, some pathologies are characterized by onsets so insidious that clues are absent until the situation is beyond retrieval. A man or woman presenting late in the course of a disease demands and deserves great efforts to heal, but the ineffectiveness of those efforts is not commonly a reflection of the quality of the care that has been given. Though physicians tend to flagellate themselves—and one another—over their inability to salvage a delayed presentation of sickness, such perceptions of personal failure are usually erroneous. Just as physicians must constantly admonish one another to seek the most subtle beginnings of disease, they must also forgive themselves when timing or circumstances frustrate their best intentions.

Experience fallacious. Though a physician's experience is, after science, his most important diagnostic and therapeutic armament, he should never allow himself to forget for a moment how it can lead him astray while caring for any one sick person, whose situation may present riddles that differ from everything else he has learned at the bedsides of so many others. The issue of individual variation in patterns of illness has been addressed by authorities as widely dissimilar in perspective as Voltaire, the French literary savant, and Claude Bernard, the first of the great modern physiologists. Voltaire, addressing the insistence of some that a sickness be given the same treatment in everyone in whom it is discovered, wrote in 1723, "What they overlook is that the diseases which afflict us are as different as the features of our faces." In his seminal mid-nineteenth-century guide to physiological research, *Introduction to Experimental Medicine*, Bernard made the same observation, based on his investigations into human biology: "A physician . . . is by no means a physician to living beings in general, not even physician to the human race, but rather, physician to a human individual, and still more physician to an individual in certain morbid conditions peculiar to himself and forming what is called his idiosyncrasy."

Experience may be misinterpreted, misremembered, and even misused, though unwittingly. Statistics, which are the recorded and combined experiences of many disease encounters, suffer from their own disabilities, including on the one hand the blending of categories of patients whose problems do not belong together, and on the other the omitting of the experiences of certain types of patients in a well-intentioned attempt to avoid precisely such inappropriate admixing. For any specific person suffering from a specific disease in a specific setting being treated in a specific environment by a specific doctor, a statistic is nothing more than a statement of relative probability.

Judgment difficult. For any bedside doctor, these two words are the distilled essence of the First Aphorism and, in fact, of all medical care; everything coming before them is merely prologue. Judgment is focused on the immediacy of the moment; the distinctive evolution of the disease in one distinctive human being leading up to that moment; the facts of the pathological process as they reveal themselves, also at that moment; the inferences drawn from the facts; the patient's emotional and biological responses to the illness; the circumstances in which the encounter occurs; and the personal background brought by the physician to this critical instant in his patient's illness—and in his own life.

Aside from considerations of experience and knowledge, not much attention has ever been paid to the final factor in the foregoing list, yet none of the others (excepting only the pathology itself) exceeds it in importance. Although a great deal has been written about the so-called doctor-patient relationship, I have encountered very little recognition of the reciprocal nature of that relationship—of its essential interdependency.

Three decades ago, I cared for an astonishingly perceptive university chaplain during the course of a protracted hospitalization, at the conclusion of which he made a number of trenchant observations about the medical team. Among his comments was one whose validity I have had plenty of opportunity to confirm since that time. "We patients," he said, "do more for you doctors than you do for us." What he was recognizing, of course, was our outsized need for the emotional rewards not only of overcoming disease but also of being healthy and strong while those who are dependent on us are diminished by their illnesses. The effect on medical care of the relationship between power and impotence is an unacknowledged thread that runs through the practice of the Art, as is our insatiable appetite for extravagant gratitude and the constant burnishing of our self-image. And these are only a few of the unstudied influences with which every linkage between doctor and patient is imbued.

There is little significant literature examining the psychology of those who choose medicine as a career, much less one or another of its specialties. Few have seriously asked, "Who are these people, and what drives them?" Whatever distancing or objectivity has been introduced into medical practice by the current array of instrumentations and intradisciplinary fragmenting, it is human beings who make the ultimate decisions about diagnosis and therapy. And they make those decisions against the background of their own emotions, needs, insecurities, strengths, strivings, and—even in these days of Freud bashing, it must be said—their own countertransferences to and identifications with those whose lives are in their hands.

Self-awareness has never been the strong suit of those who choose to become doctors. When so much fuel is readily available for stoking the fires of ego, there is little inclination to apply it in raising the candlepower of the searching light that might illumine the inner man or woman. I would venture to guess that the percentage of unexamined lives in my profession is shockingly high. Yet the rewards of identifying and facing one's own motivations and tremblings are enormous. I refer here not to some idealized hope of overcoming what is undesirable in ourselves but rather to the more practical wish that physicians might pursue self-knowledge with a distinctly clinical aim in mind: to help us understand what can be brought to consciousness about why we incline one way or another in the choice of pathways along which we send our patients. Judgment is difficult enough without adding to the problem by further obscuring the dimly recognized or unspoken motives that may influence it. As the aphorism says, the

Art is long, and there is little we are able to do about the shortness of our own lives. But we can deepen our understanding of ourselves, and in this way deepen our ability to help our patients, and add breadth to the value of our days.

Doctors expect a great deal of themselves. Patients expect a great deal of their doctors. As has been true since the time of Hippocrates, some of those expectations are unrealistic, while others might best be met by a more frequent inward focus, a bit more understanding of one another, and a mutual recognition of what is possible and what is not. This, I believe, is the ultimate message in the First Aphorism and the reason it will always be the whole law of medicine. We should enjoin ourselves—doctors and patients alike—to go and study it.

NARCISSUS LOOKS INTO
THE LABORATORY

Among the many ancient Greek medical writings that scholars of an earlier generation credited to Hippocrates, there is a particularly interesting essay that deals with the education of a physician. The brief length of "Law" —only five paragraphs—and certain of its trenchant observations, caused one translator to call it a "quaint little piece" and voice regret that "it has strangely been neglected by scholars." His concern was no doubt based on the fact that this particular gem contains more good sense per line than any of the approximately sixty treatises once thought to have been written by the Father of Medicine himself.

Some of the statements in "Law" are more aphoristic than the vast majority of those in *The Aphorisms* and exceed them in universality. And as for being timeless—well, try this one, about time itself: "It is time which imparts strength to all things and brings them to maturity." I found myself thinking about just this statement one day a few years ago while reading a newspaper account of yet another triumph in the world of molecular biology, this one being page-one-headlined by an exuberant *New York Times*: "In Big Advance in Cloning, Biologists Create 50 Mice."

Imagine that—the biologist as creator! Or, perhaps before too long, as Creator.

Not only did the researchers "churn out clones of adult mice," announced the *Times*, but they even went so far as to make clones of clones. One authority at Princeton University (to whom the article refers as a "mouse geneticist") "described the speed at which the cloning had progressed as breathtaking." He went further: "'Absolutely,' he said, 'we're going to have cloning of humans.'" According to the mouse expert, even the safeguards of strict scientific protocol and the delay required to perfect the technique in monkeys would not prevent in vitro fertilization clinics from being able to add human cloning to their bag of tricks within a dazzlingly short period of time.

It's not enough that we are plunging pell-mell toward cloning one another. Even the genetic enhancement of laboratory-crafted people is now being talked about. This would mean quite a bit more than the current therapeutic aims of introducing genes into patients to fight or ward off disease or of cloning for the purposes of tissue and organ transplantation. Changes are now being considered that would improve the very germplasm, the permanent heredity, of these "created" clones. Traits thus made inherent would be potentially transferable to every succeeding generation. This goes beyond fantasizing about Bionic Man to conjuring up the dream of Designer Man.

The velocity of our head-over-heels rush to clinical fulfillment comes into perspective when we recall that little more than a decade has passed since the newborn Dolly first made those appealing sheep's eyes at the television cameras in July 1996. At that time, no serious scientist believed that an attempt to reproduce the feat in humans would take place within a reasonable period. Now there seems, at least in the minds of some, not much doubt that the technological moment at which it will be possible to create a human embryo is almost at hand.

Meanwhile, other researchers are less concerned with crafting an improved version of the present generation for transmission into the next than with playing around with a project that has been dear to mankind's heart ever since our species first made its appearance in dim prehistory. For these scientists, it is not sufficient to clone our bettered selves into interminable generations; they are experimenting with techniques that might have the potential to make some members of our generation themselves interminable. Their goal is the lengthening of life beyond any span that clinical and public health advances (which have already added some thirty-five years to our life expectancy during the century just passed) might anticipate. What they are talking about now is an increase not only in expectancy but in the very life span granted by nature and evolution to our and every other species.

Noting that a structure found at the end of the DNA molecule, called a telomere, decreases in size each time a cell divides, these researchers have been working with a gene that codes for the enzyme telomerase. Telomerase has the ability to maintain or even increase the length of the telomere. In the laboratory, such manipulation has resulted in a marked increase in the number of times a cell can divide before dying. As recently as a dozen years ago, responsible molecular biologists scoffed at the idea that this work could accomplish such things, but no longer. Telomerase is now a hot research topic.

There is something just a bit scary about the way researchers describe what they see in their experiments. They say the cells are *rejuvenated*, a word reminiscent of the age-old search for a source of renewed vigor that culminated during the early twentieth century in the "magical" effects of monkey gland extracts and other such nostrums for perpetuating youth.

Not only would some of the current rush to fruition have been deemed absurdly futuristic only a decade ago, but the often overheated media have flavored their reports of it with the promise of imminent wondrous applications to human happiness. I discovered my favorite in the selfsame *New York Times*, reporting telomerase's extension of cellular reproductive lines with a detailed story, in the lead paragraph of which was posed a tantalizing question: "If cells can be made to live indefinitely, can people be made immortal?" The large headline over the article read, "Longevity's New Lease on Life." Can anyone be blamed for believing that this fantasy is close to becoming reality?

The media are not without reason for enthusiasm. Daring statements are being made by otherwise cautious scientists about the implications of their work. As one after another of nature's hitherto closely guarded secrets is revealed by their relentless ingenuity, researchers have begun to allow themselves to think the previously unthinkable.

Some of their rumination, like that of the mouse geneticist, is public. As in his case, it generally takes the form of pithy quotes delivered over telephone lines in response to questing science writers, who then rush them into print for immediate consumption by a public eager to believe that a New Jerusalem of health and longevity is at hand. Perhaps egged on by their recently acquired prophetic image, many biomedical scientists have abandoned the restraint that has long characterized their breed. To the usual unbounded zeal for the next research step has been added a less usual unbounded zeal for the immediacy of clinical use. Because of a few awe-inspiring discoveries, many ordinary citizens have changed their opinion about how far we dare to look ahead and how fast we dare to go. Caught up in the infectious excitement of biomedical science and its commentators, we seem to have forgotten about the leavening effect of time's passage—and the maturity it can bring.

Our society has become very much like an overstimulated child. Perhaps such an analogy can be taken even further. The by-products of biomedicine's brilliance have rubbed off on all of us, even those without the training or background to grasp fully the factual basis of the advances. The kind of child our society resembles just now is one whose intelligence far exceeds his maturity. Every teacher and every parent knows what a formula for disaster that can be. Among some of the scientists themselves, the brilliance-to-maturity ratio may be strikingly higher than among the general population, and not only because they tend to be smarter than the rest of us.

This might be the time to do just what wise teachers do when faced with such a situation in the classroom: a child whose intellectual attainments far outstrip his ability to deal with the consequences of being so smart, a child who is likely, therefore, to make mistakes in using his genius that will ultimately harm himself and others. What a wise teacher does with such a child is not to promote him to the next grade when the school year ends. The child stays where he is until his social abilities catch up to his brainpower. Years ago, it was the custom to push such brilliant kids forward rapidly through the grades, but the price—in psychological illness and even breakdowns—proved to be very high. Too many of these bright youngsters never fulfilled the promise of their intellectual gifts because they were not given the time to mature. Had they been kept back, they would have been allowed to grow up enough to comprehend what might happen as a result of their genius.

What I am suggesting here is a brake on the application of technologies whose consequences we can at present only begin to contemplate. For the first time in the annals of scientific research, we are faced with discoveries whose implications to society go far beyond the community of researchers, physicians, and those patients who would be directly involved. We may have reached the point where we can no longer afford to permit scientists alone to determine how far to carry the applications of their work. Some might even suggest that the *direction* of research, too, should be influenced by open discussion in our society. Though most of us would be reluctant to take such a position, the borderline between the basic science laboratory and the laboratory for product development has become so obscure that even such a radical proposition might one day need to be entertained.

But regardless of the stance taken in such matters, one obvious truth must be acknowledged: when an entire society is to be affected, the entire informed society should participate in the decisions. The society should slow down and give itself time to think, time to confer, time to mature.

The federal government has shown signs of understanding the present dilemma. In 1995, President Clinton formed the National Bioethics Advisory Commission to deal with the kinds of issues raised by the new branches of research. In what may prove to be its most significant decision, this panel—composed of representatives from the fields of medicine, nursing, religion, law, ethics, industry, education, and health advocacy—did in effect decide to keep the child back a grade by supporting the president's planned moratorium on the use of federal funds to attempt human cloning. In its ninety days of deliberation, during which the commission heard testimony from a cross section of informed societal interests, it came down on the side of banning application, while supporting the need for continuing research. Implicit in its recommendations are two guiding and interrelated notions: first, although we have knowledge aplenty, there would be no benefit—even if it were practically possible—in ceasing to pursue even more knowledge; second, knowledge without wisdom is a clear and present danger. The members of the commission did not have to add the lesson of "Law," that wisdom comes only with maturity and maturity comes only with time.

Since then, the commission's current equivalent—the Bush-appointed President's Council on Bioethics—has, under two successive chairmen noted for their conservative positions on such matters, continued the ban. Unfortunately, however, the council has gone much further than the great majority of scientists and the general public deem appropriate, including the promulgation of restrictions on stem cell research. But in making a decision with implications far beyond the bounds of reasonable prudence, the administration has willy-nilly called public attention to the complexities that arise when the authority of government is mistaken for the voice of society itself.

All of this government tinkering illustrates the urgency of informed societal involvement. But unlike the situation of stem cell research, the usual problem is the obverse: Federal funds are not infrequently granted to research efforts without sufficient regard to the long-term social or ethical implications of new discovery. Our society should at least pause briefly to think about its motivations for plunging forward without due consideration of the range of possible consequences or of the immediate financial cost of the research in a time of limited resources. The great advances in the real health of humanity in the past hundred years—particularly when evaluated in the perspective of our entire planet—have occurred more as the result of such preventive measures as immunization, personal cleanliness, water purification, proper diet, and other public health efforts than from any application, except antibiotics and perhaps improvements in cardiac care, of the technologies of cure to individual patients. These preventive measures—and not surgery, pharmacology, molecular biology, or the therapies given in hospitals—are the primary reason for our vastly improved life expectancy. It is health, after all, that should concern us. And it should concern us far more than the mere desire to perpetuate ourselves.

Prevention and early diagnosis are more direct routes to health and a good quality of life than any stratagem yet devised, or likely to be devised, in our lifetimes. As long as resources are finite, as they always will be, we would do well not to abandon the wisdom that has stood us in such good stead in the past. The magnificences served up daily by the molecular biologists may exhilarate us, but our real goal should not be the satisfaction of the egocentricity within each of us. To this end, we need to review not only our headlong dash into the arms of the researchers but our priorities as well.

The search for wisdom is always fraught with danger, but those inherent in the present situation arise from the very fabric of human character. After all, who among us has not occasionally, or more than occasionally, cherished the notion that we might live forever, or that we might stay young far beyond our years, or that we might even continue to exist in the form of a descendant who is, at least genetically, our duplicate? For some, these are more than just notions—they are a prevailing philosophy of life, even an obsession. Maybe this is why, when practical applications are only the glib predictions of overzealous researchers, keen votaries have uncritically hailed the future of genetic studies that might hold some possibility of these outcomes.

The prevailing mood of our time is self-absorption and its natural extension, narcissism. Manifestations are everywhere apparent: the youth culture; the huge market in cosmetic surgery; the entire cult of "personal fulfillment"; the so-called human potential movement; the outsize emphasis on the individual as opposed to the cultural group and even the family; the popularity of new drugs to grow new hair or build new erections; and, finally, the very situation I am addressing here—the possibility that research in genetics will put us on the road toward eternal life. In pursuing vanity, far too many of us have simply lost hold of our senses. There has never been a period in human history during which the creed of self-indulgence has found so many apostles.

If there exists a single characteristic that unifies all self-absorption and vanity, it surely must be foolishness. Knowing lots of things does not make us any less foolish. Mere information is only the beginning of knowledge, and even knowledge does not of itself lead to maturity, nor does it guarantee good judgment. We need to grow up a lot more as a society before we are ready to play with the new toys being so efficiently made for us by the precocious scientists. Growing up takes time and reflection. T. S. Eliot reminds us that we have paid a high price for the compulsion to accelerate the engines of our existence:

> Where is the Life we have lost in living?
> Where is the wisdom we have lost in knowledge?
> Where is the knowledge we have lost in information?

THE MEDICAL SCHOOL
AND THE UNIVERSITY

The facade of one of the two outward-facing wings of the Yale School of Medicine bears an Ozymandian inscription: INSTITUTE OF HUMAN RELATIONS. As Shelley told us, that great conquerer's "shattered visage" and "vast and trunkless legs of stone" were all that was left of the lofty claims of a forgotten era, and so it is with the building's name. Both in the ancient suzerainty of Ozymandias and at Yale, "nothing beside remains" of a powerful leader's dream, except those few traces proclaiming a majesty that lived for a brief time and today exists in the memory of almost no one.

Only rarely does a passing student or visitor comment on the imposing words chiseled into the medical school's granite front or wonder that one wing of this grand building should be dedicated to a concept that seems not only abstruse but also unrelated to the mission of a modern medical school. What, precisely, could be meant by "Institute of Human Relations"? What might have been the intention of its founder, and what could the inscription have to do with the teaching or practice of medicine?

In fact, the founding of the Institute of Human Relations in 1929 was perhaps the most ambitious step ever taken toward the idealistic goal of creating a firm bond of unity between a medical school and the rest of its university—a bond so firm that students and faculties of both would intermingle, exchange ideas, and join in projects for the betterment of academic life and of humankind in general. It was the bold idea of a bold man.

When Milton Winternitz arrived at Yale from Johns Hopkins as professor of pathology in 1917, the medical school was at a low point in its fortunes and reputation. Within three years Winternitz had exerted such a dynamic and visionary influence on the school's affairs that he was elected dean. Described by colleagues as "an intense fountainhead of energy, an inexhaustible generator of ideas and constant stimulator of the imagination"—and more vividly by Yale's president, James Rowland Angell, as "that steam engine in pants"—Winternitz was determined to bring the medical school closer to the university in academic standards, in intellectual spirit, and in educational philosophy. He raised standards for admission and for faculty recruitment; redesigned the curriculum to allow students to indulge their research, clinical, and even humanistic interests in a variety of ways; and organized the various medical specialties into academic departments. In establishing his conviction that medical students should be seen as graduate students whose intellectual milieu is the entire campus, he saw to it that young people from various disciplines in the Yale community intermingled in the classroom.

To Winternitz, medicine was a social science. Its primary concerns had traditionally been with sick organs, but he saw the proper role of a medical school as the study of the whole man living in a social and economic environment. To understand disease, one had to understand health and the conditions that affect it. In this Winternitz was a disciple of the great nineteenth-century German pathologist Rudolf Virchow, who believed that the health of an individual is largely determined by the socioeconomic conditions under which he lives. Virchow was the greatest microscopic pathologist of his age (known, in fact, as "the Pope of German medicine"), but he was also the greatest proponent of what he called the "humanistic" view of patients, individually and collectively. As a scientist, Virchow defined humanism as "the scientific knowledge of the manifold and various relations of the thoughtful individual person to the ever-changing world."

Though separated by culture, generation, and geography, Winternitz and Virchow had much in common. They were both small, wiry men who were not physically prepossessing. Capable of enormous amounts of work, both were martinet-like in the demands they made on themselves and others, to the point that they were feared or disliked by many colleagues and students even as they were held in near-universal awe as scientists and leaders in their profession. Both became legends in their institutions and their disciplines.

It seemed obvious to Winternitz that the only way to achieve his objectives was to meld his school into the general academic life around it—a goal that had never been attained since medical faculties first became parts of greater teaching institutions in Montpellier, Paris, and Bologna in the early thirteenth century. On the continent of Europe, those three great shrines of learning had spawned a tradition that the education of physicians was to be conducted in the university; but medical faculties had remained, for the most part, quite separate from the activities of the other intellectual disciplines that grew up over the centuries. In England, in fact, the best medical teaching was found at independent schools that had been established in large hospitals. In all countries the great majority of physicians, and especially surgeons, were educated by some form of apprenticeship to an established practitioner, from whom they learned the rudiments of care via a nonsystem that might be thought of as on-the-job training. In time, guildlike societies accorded some form of certification to the best-trained and most capable doctors, but until well into the nineteenth century the ordinary citizen was unlikely to be treated by someone whose skills had been evaluated by a formal body of experts.

The situation in North America emerged from a mix of these backgrounds. Until the establishment of a medical school at the University of Pennsylvania in 1765, it was impossible to obtain the MD degree in the Western Hemisphere. Young men traveled to various European schools to study medicine; the most popular institution—and the one that most influenced the development of an American system—was the University of Edinburgh. But such students were relatively few. Of twelve hundred physicians who served in the colonial army during the Revolutionary War, only a hundred had medical degrees. The rest had been trained in the apprenticeship system. Even by 1800, only two other American medical schools had been established—at King's College (now Columbia University) and Harvard.

At this point the American entrepreneurial spirit made itself felt. Responding to the need for formal medical training, physicians began to open private "proprietary" schools, which provided a half-dozen lectures per day supplemented by assigned readings in standard texts. Between 1810 and 1876, no fewer than seventy-three new schools were founded. Though some were nominally associated with a university, the great majority were doctor-owned and profit-driven. The mass teaching was often so poor that faculty members augmented their income by giving private instruction, individually or in small groups, to those who could afford it. Even after the middle of the nineteenth century, when scientific research had become an important part of European medical thought, none but the most rudimentary forms of laboratory equipment could be found in such schools—and even then in only a few of them.

A mere handful of the approximately fifty university-affiliated medical schools in the United States were able to attain a higher level of teaching and bedside instruction than the norm. An American doctor might fill the gaps in his education by "walking the wards" and taking courses in a European clinic. The popularity of Parisian hospitals in the early part of the century was superseded by that of German-speaking schools after about 1860. In the two decades before 1900, a number of young Americans took part in research directed by leading German scientists. Imbued with the spirit of what their mentors called *Lehrfreiheit und Lernfreiheit* (best translated as academic freedom, a notion that grew out of the rebellions of 1848), they chafed against the straitjacketed ways in which medicine was being taught in their native land. There arose a cadre of leaders in the profession who were concerned about the generally low level of the American system of medical education, and about its restrictions on freedom of thought.

Since its founding in 1847, the American Medical Association had been deeply concerned about the poor training of most physicians. In 1906 its Council on Medical Education conducted a study of all of the nation's medical schools.

Measured by criteria that the council considered the highest university standard, the entire system was shown to be in disarray. Only the recently founded Johns Hopkins Medical School, based entirely on the German model of a research university with high achievement by both faculty and students, provided the academic atmosphere that was thought essential if American physicians were to take their place among the world's most accomplished in science and clinical care.

The well-funded Carnegie Foundation for the Advancement of Teaching, established a year earlier, was concerned with the same problem. In 1908, its directors chose an experienced educator, Abraham Flexner, to carry out an exhaustive study of the nation's 155 medical schools, using the Johns Hopkins model and the council's advice to define the criteria of excellence. Flexner's findings were as appalling as the AMA's. His 1910 report, now considered a classic in the literature of medicine (and of education), contained explicit recommendations that would so transform American medical schools that within a few decades they would be recognized as the best in the world.

Flexner's most fundamental thesis, perhaps, was his correct insistence that medicine must be taught and practiced on a scientific basis. This, he stated, "gives an undoubted advantage to the university medical departments." The success of Johns Hopkins had proved this. Hopkins was the perfect example of a school based on the principle of scientific medicine and the necessity that its faculty be intensely committed to research. The details of the Hopkins system became the foundation on which medical schools would remodel themselves as faculties within a university. The proprietary schools rapidly disappeared.

In their understandable eagerness to view their university affiliation as the foundation of a scientific approach to medical thought, the leaders of American medicine committed themselves to a course of action that would forever link education to research. In essence, they had made an irrevocable decision: the educational institution was also to be a research institution. A faculty dedicated to one would henceforth have to be dedicated to both. Never mind that the skills and personal qualities required in the two arenas were quite different; never mind that approximately half the faculty would, in addition, have to provide exemplary clinical care to patients, adding yet a third necessary talent to their already-difficult responsibilities.

Instead of a chair, a medical professor would occupy a seat that has since become notorious for its unsteadiness: the now-famous three-legged stool of excellence in teaching, research, and clinical work. Sitting on it is akin to remaining mounted on three spirited horses at once: the rider is likely to find himself galloping furiously in all directions.

Of all the manifold problems afflicting the modern medical school, one of the most serious and least frequently addressed is the inherent inconsistency among its several aims. As admirable as each aim may be by itself, only a rare faculty can meet the highest standards in each. For professors in clinical disciplines such as internal medicine, surgery, and pediatrics, the problem has been aggravated in recent years by the necessity of increasing the patient population in order to guarantee the financial solvency of their departments.

If one is a clinician whose notion of a medical school is that it should be a place where young people come to learn how to take care of the sick, the most fundamental difficulty arises from the primacy of research. Since the 1960s, the level of medical investigation has become increasingly sophisticated, as the requirements of molecular and genetic studies have demanded an ever-more-meticulous understanding of laboratory and interpretive methodologies. Nowadays even clinical research is likely to involve a deep knowledge of such disciplines as statistics and epidemiology. With each passing decade, both students and faculty have become more engrossed in such laboratory and clinical studies. The decision to link education to research has evolved—because there are only so many hours in a day and only so many days in a four-year course—into the decision that a medical school should be a highly specialized and compartmentalized institution. Some have even begun to characterize it as a trade school. The ideal of a liberal permeation by the wider university now seems more remote than ever.

Medical schools rarely promote teachers for teaching well or for caring for (or even about) the sick. Their prestige generally rests on the number of NIH and foundation grants they receive and the nationally renowned scientists who grace their research wings. In the preclinical sciences, such as molecular biology, genetics, and immunology, instruction often involves an overemphasis on the particular part of the field in which the teacher is working, and frequently on his or her own pet interests. Even in such seemingly "bedside" disciplines as surgery and internal medicine, the research these days is less likely to apply to direct patient care than to molecular-level phenomena. That's where the big discoveries, the big accolades, and the big bucks are.

Milton Winternitz had already recognized the oncoming tide of these phenomena in the 1920s. A distinguished scientist himself, he feared the future emphasis on laboratory science that he saw as engulfing the primary mission of the medical school. To stem it—to turn medicine's attention back to the sick patient in the hospital bed—he conceived of the Institute of Human Relations, a haven from academic medicine's determination to transform itself into an investigational and technological enterprise. There he would bring to bear all the forces of sociology, psychology, economics, industry, law, government, education, and public health, so that individual patients might be studied and treated as whole persons. No longer would Yale be content to turn out the kind of physician that Winternitz scorned as a mere "doctor-technician."

One can only guess how far the program might have gone. The aims were high; the inclusion of such disciplines as literature, philosophy, and history might have been the next step. As Winternitz saw it, the fragmentation of medical education would begin to break down, barriers between disciplines would crumble, and the increasing distance between doctor and patient would be narrowed. The Institute of Human Relations would be truly humane.

Winternitz recruited many powerful people in the university to his side. They traveled throughout the country to explain the institute's plans to alumni and civic groups. Seven and a half million dollars were donated, the building rose, and the facade was proudly inscribed with those seemingly indelible words. The dedication took place on May 9, 1931. A distinguished faculty had been gathered from various parts of the university, all committed to a collective effort.

It was not to be. Almost as soon as it started, the grand scheme began falling to pieces. Collaborators did not collaborate, slipping back instead into the old fragmentation; the departments of the medical school—always skeptical of diverting themselves into areas they saw as "soft"—kept themselves aloof; resentments arose over Winternitz's attempts to control space allocation and, increasingly, over what was perceived as his dictatorial attitude toward the entire enterprise. Within a few years, the Institute of Human Relations was no more. The faculty returned to its own parochial interests. Gone the way of the empire of Ozymandias, the great dream that a medical school could be integrated into the humanistic endeavor of a university had vanished.

It needs to be revived. The problems Winternitz was attempting to solve have become more urgent than they were seventy years ago. The expanding "scientization" of medicine has led, more and more, to the dehumanization of medicine. It is time once again to address the role of medical education in dealing with "the manifold and various relations of the thoughtful individual person to the ever-changing world." Unless the liberating influence of the entire university can be brought to bear, we in the medical profession will continue to deserve—now more than ever—the pejorative description of "doctor-technicians," better at curing than caring, better at understanding pathology than understanding the distressed men and women who come to us to be healed.

THE TRUE HEALERS

Men are men before they are lawyers, or physicians, or merchants, or manufacturers; and if you make them capable and sensible men, they will make themselves capable and sensitive lawyers or physicians. What professional men should carry away with them from an University, is not professional knowledge, but that which should direct the use of their professional knowledge, and bring the light of general culture to illuminate the technicalities of a general pursuit.

JOHN STUART MILL
INAUGURAL ADDRESS AS RECTOR OF
ST. ANDREW'S UNIVERSITY, 1867

Training is not the same as education. When the Carnegie Foundation's Abraham Flexner published his incisive critique of American medical schools in 1910, he properly issued the crucial dictum that the teaching of medicine must be founded upon a strong basis of science. Without this foundation, a physician could not possibly understand the workings and disabilities of the human body, which were being so rapidly elucidated in many European and a few American research laboratories. It was apparent to Flexner and to everyone who read his report that science is best taught in a university atmosphere.

One of Flexner's most cogent arguments for teaching science under university auspices was his concern that it would otherwise not be understood in its full context. He feared that if subjects such as bacteriology and pathology were compartmentalized in order to train students specifically for medical practice, future doctors would not acquire the true appreciation of the broad range of human biology that physicians needed if they were to understand the setting in which their patients became ill. "Both subjects," wrote Flexner, "are, indeed, full-grown biological sciences—university subjects, capable of cultivation only in special laboratories, closely affiliated with general biology and chemistry."

Flexner cared not only about what he called "curative medicine" but also about prevention, which he believed to be possible only with a keen knowledge of the conditions in which disease arises. In an almost lyrical passage, he presented his idealized image of an educational experience from which "emerges the young physician, equipped with sound views as to the nature, causation, spread, prevention, and cure of disease, and with an exalted conception of his own duty to promote social conditions that conduce to physical well-being."

Flexner was using "exalted" not in today's ironic sense of "exaggerated" but, quite precisely, to mean "lofty" or "sublime." The same ideas had been expressed by the social reformer and pathologist Rudolf Virchow in the nineteenth century; they would be among the foundation stones used by Milton Winternitz to build the Institute of Human Relations at Yale, described in the foregoing chapter. Flexner thus recognized that "the practitioner deals with facts of two categories. Chemistry, physics, biology enable him to apprehend one set; he needs a different apperceptive and appreciative apparatus to deal with other, more subtle elements. Specific preparation is in this direction much more difficult; one must rely for the requisite insight and sympathy on a varied and enlarging cultural experience. Such enlargement of the physician's horizon is otherwise important, for scientific progress has greatly modified his ethical responsibility. . . . It goes without saying that this type of doctor is first of all an educated man."

This brief passage was the only part of Flexner's 346-page report in which he made any mention of the "varied and enlarging cultural experience" that he considered so important to the education of physicians. His few words on the subject were forgotten in the well-justified rush to implement his outpouring of critical recommendations. Influenced by Flexner's report, medical schools sought close affiliations with hospitals, full-time faculty members began to replace teachers who had divided their time between the school and their lucrative private practices, and—most important to the entire scheme's success—

medical teaching became fully established on the firm foundation of university-based science. Moreover, research contributions became a prime criterion in recruiting new faculty.

The Flexner Report, as it became known, outlined the steps that would raise American medical education to world leadership. Among the consequences of the report was the creation of an atmosphere for research and clinical excellence that made the United States preeminent not only in biomedical discovery but also in the treatment of disease. The growth of American university medical centers has been one of the most remarkable phenomena in the history of science and education. These citadels of medicine are civic enterprises unto themselves—scientific, economic, and social enterprises that have, over the years, taken on or been beset by such a wide range of challenges that they are now fraught with as many problems as solutions.

Too often forgotten today is the simple fact that all the vastness and chaotic intellectual ferment of the modern academic medical center have grown out of attempts to teach individual students how to care for the sick. Yet more often than not, the pedagogical mission of our schools has been lost in the thicket of undertakings that now consume the faculty and staff. The mood of unrelenting growth of the four decades since the 1960s is epitomized in a single sentence from a newsletter sent only a few years ago to faculty members at one giant institution that is widely recognized as being among the nation's finest. The dean of this medical school announced an innovation: "This spring we created the new position of deputy dean for education, formally placing the teaching mission on a par with research and clinical affairs."

And high time, wouldn't you say? No doubt the school's action reflected a belated recognition of a situation spawned by the tumultuous atmosphere in which researchers and clinicians make headlong leaps toward ever-greater achievements. But one wonders whether the dean appreciated the irony of his announcement. In essence he was admitting that the stupendous growth of the other areas in which his institution is involved had subverted the school's basic purpose.

He also implied something more: that until now, no leader of his institution had considered the oversight of its primary mission—

education—to be an especially important function, at least as compared with the oversight of research and clinical affairs. This surprising omission has been facilitated by a premise well known to anyone involved with the extraordinary young people now studying at American medical schools: put them in close proximity to excellent scientific clinicians and researchers and they will learn, willy-nilly, how to be excellent scientific clinicians and researchers—even when there is little or no formal teaching. They do learn, by a sort of on-the-job training. But what students are not likely to acquire from the technologically minded men and women who nowadays represent the great majority of the faculty of our best medical schools is the Flexnerian "different apperceptive and appreciative apparatus to deal with other, more subtle elements," specifically those elements that require "a varied and enlarging cultural experience." That "enlargement of the physician's horizon," as Flexner nicely put it, "is much more difficult."

By insisting that a doctor should first of all be "an educated man," Flexner meant that those treating the sick must commit themselves to caring for the whole man or woman, not just his or her pathology. The true healer should have a wide knowledge of the culture in which he and his patients live and a deep understanding of the many varieties of the human condition. Though they can undoubtedly obtain some of this awareness at the bedside, today's doctors in training would greatly expand and enrich their limited interactions with patients if they came to them armed with a liberal education and a background in humanistic thought. It is not too much to ask that a physician's learning should encompass an overview of the entire range of our civilization's cultural development and a reasonably detailed knowledge of certain aspects of it. The wisdom of any of us is circumscribed by our relatively limited experience of life. We expand it by studying literature, history, philosophy, and the evolution and beliefs of societies not our own.

The profession's educators have on occasion shown evidence of understanding this and of trying to do something about it. Some have shouted vainly from the depths of the dense and tangled growth that is today's academic medical center. Others have formally protested within their professional organizations, demanding change. It is good to know that nonscience majors are now being admitted to medical schools at the same rate as their peers who have spent four undergraduate years absorbed in laboratories and measurements; that there has been a significant increase in the number of medical schools that offer (and sometimes even require) courses in literature, ethics, and medical history; that many schools now have full-time chaplains with whom students can engage not only for counsel but also for discussion and debate; that the recent upsurge in attention to end-of-life care has served to remind many doctors of their pastoral role in guiding patients (and themselves) through the trials of death as well as the triumphs of cure.

But these efforts don't yet suffice. As long ago as 1984, the Association of American Medical Colleges published a study called "Physicians for the 21st Century," in which can be found the much overlooked recommendation that "each medical school campus have at least one full-time humanist to lead research in these areas and to act as a catalyst and liaison with other course directors to ensure that humanities materials are integrated into the curriculum." Other bodies have been making similar suggestions for at least the past four decades, to little avail. In 1989 the American College of Surgeons (yes, surgeons) devoted an entire issue of its quarterly *Bulletin* to the importance of knowledge of the humanities. The result of all the official nudging is that some schools do have "at least one full-time humanist"; many, however, do not. The scattered courses in humanistic studies now available in so many institutions are rarely "integrated into the curriculum," and, in any event, they are infrequently attended by any but first- and second-year students. Satisfying the demands of the science so vigorously advocated by Flexner has gone well past its required endpoint, but his comments about the importance of the "more subtle elements" are in large part neglected or given mere lip service. There is so much overkill in the teaching of basic biomedical science and clinical techniques in today's academic medical centers that little or no time remains in the curriculum for the development of the physician's wholeness, or for the recognition of each patient's uniqueness. Milton

Winternitz's scornful term "doctor-technician" seems to have become the ideal of medical training.

It's long past time to reverse the process by which the teaching of healing became the teaching of biomedicine. Like other wars, turf wars for the student's time and attention are won by those with the most powerful armaments and the most committed soldiers and leaders. As things now stand, the case for humanistic studies cannot be effectively argued at meetings of curriculum committees; nor can any battles be won by individual advocates, no matter how high their level of passion or how clearly right their cause. What's required in any school is a fully equipped army with a dedicated general staff to counteract the forceful encroachments of those who now overwhelm the four-year schedule with science and technology. By this I mean that it is no longer enough to make pious recommendations about the place of the humanities in the curriculum. Radical action is required. Only by creating a fully staffed and well-funded department of humanities in medicine will a school fulfill the proclaimed commitment of such bodies as the Association of American Medical Colleges and the American College of Surgeons.

The creation of such a unit would go beyond teaching and research. It would be a statement and symbol of the importance that medical educators attach to the development of complete physicians. The presence of a strong department of medical humanities would tell students that mastering genetics, molecular biology, or neurosurgery is not considered a greater good than learning to be a real doctor. It behooves foundations and funding agencies to see the value in such endeavors and to commit resources of as much as ten million dollars (or more) per school to change a situation that so many foundations and agencies have decried. When the Department of Medical Humanities of my alma mater is as powerful and highly regarded as its Department of Pathology, we will be turning out the kinds of physicians that Flexner and Winternitz—and, more than a century ago, Virchow—dreamed of.

Ten million dollars is a lot of money. Multiply it by our nation's 124 medical schools, and it becomes a practical impossibility. Nor am I foolish enough to think that my proposal will necessarily achieve its intended purpose. Certain pitfalls are easy to see, and as in all enormous undertakings, there will be others that cannot yet be imagined. But should any so-disposed foundation directors or philanthropic billionaires be reading this, my suggestion would be to choose three to five schools of different types and to begin by establishing fully staffed and strong humanities departments at those institutions, in a sense as pilot projects. If they prove successful, similar programs might be introduced elsewhere.

In 1996, Anne Fadiman published a notable book titled *The Spirit Catches You and You Fall Down*. It describes a cultural clash between the values and practices of American medicine and those of newly arrived Laotian immigrants of the Hmong tribe. At the center of the story is a young girl who is seriously damaged by a series of misunderstandings about a course of treatment for epilepsy. The doctors involved could not have been better trained or better intentioned. As Fadiman put it, they were excellent physicians but imperfect healers. I don't know how to make doctors perfect, but at least we can provide them with an education that will help them to heal, not merely to cure.

PUMPING IRON

The Roman satirist Juvenal counseled his readers that the labors of Hercules are to be preferred to soft cushions and great feasts. One should pray for *mens sana in corpore sano*, he advised, rather than for a life of indolence. A millennium and a half later, John Locke appropriated that aphorism, "A sound mind in a sound body," in his celebrated *Some Thoughts Concerning Education*, and since then it has been a proclaimed theme for nearly every generation of teachers.

But like youth, which we all agree should not be wasted on the young, the admonition of the poet and the philosopher needs to be snatched up by people of all ages. Those of us who are getting on in years, in particular, should snatch it up and run with it—literally. In recent years, study after study has shown that exercise of mind and body is the key not only to what Locke called "a happy state in this world" but to increased longevity and prolonged independence. Readers of daily newspapers have seen the reports of leading research groups confirming that vigorous activity by middle-aged or older people prevents or at least significantly lessens loss of muscle strength and bone density, which are responsible for so much disability and even disease.

As for intellectual capacity, it is by now well known that the best way to maintain mental function is to exercise it. Or, as Oliver Wendell Holmes famously put it, "Men do not quit playing because they grow old; they grow old because they quit playing." This is as true for the brain and nerves as it is for bones and muscles. The proficiency of the synapse, where an impulse is transmitted from one nerve cell to another, is strengthened by frequent use. It retains its capacity to change, even to become more effective, throughout life.

Recent studies hint at the possibility that this may also be true of the nerve cells themselves. Their ability to generate impulses—what neuroscientists call "electrogenicity"—appears to respond to changes in input. The electrogenic machinery can apparently be remodeled, and patterns of electrical activity altered, depending on the kind and frequency of stimuli that reach the cell. So keep reading. You may be strengthening your synapses and building your electrogenicity.

All this sophisticated talk adds up to no more than the advice that was so often proclaimed by the late syndicated sage Ann Landers: "Use it or lose it." And it certainly confirms everyone's daily observations. Simply put, active people remain active. Though it is comforting to have it confirmed by Landers, by laboratories, and by the learned, we have all known for a very long time that the key to productivity is productivity.

What we have not known are the details. At first gradually, and now with increasing velocity, not only scientists but fitness experts, too, are learning the specifics of just what is required to preserve ourselves— if not necessarily to a greater age, at least to one less encumbered by the debilities that too often characterize the final years of life. Even should "using it" not succeed in prolonging our days, vigorous activity of mind and muscle is the secret of better aging, or what the gerontologists call "compression of morbidity." By this they mean the goal of so decreasing the frequency of sickness and disability in the elderly that their period of decline is much shortened. The long-range goal is to make the graph of the approach to life's termination resemble a horizontal line followed by a more or less perpendicular drop-off near the end, rather than a gradually downward-sloping curve to the grave, even if the date of the endpoint proves to be unchangeable.

As for that endpoint date, there is, of course, abundant evidence, both anecdotal and statistical, of the beneficial effect of exercise on life expectancy, and it has been accumulating for a long time. Readers of this book might find one reported study of particular interest because it deals with a cohort of subjects very well studied for an extensive period. A long-term evaluation of fifty-two thousand male graduates of Harvard College and the University of Pennsylvania has shown that alumni between the ages of thirty-five and seventy-four who over the years expended at least two thousand calories per week in vigorous activities had a risk of cardiovascular disease and death that was 25 percent lower than that of less active men. Not only that, but men who took up an active life long after college did better than former student athletes who had quit in middle age. Couch potatoes should note the jock-image titles of both the article and the professional publication in which it was printed: "A Natural History of Athleticism, Health and Longevity," in the *Journal of Sports Sciences.*

Though the link between exercise and longevity may not be news, only recently has loss of muscle strength been recognized as a major element in causing the disabilities that overtake us as we get older. The greater the age, the greater the contribution of frailty, until it—and not any named disease—becomes the single most important determinant of quality of life. In a paper published in *Science* in October 1997, a team of Dutch researchers reported that their studies had convinced them that "in the oldest old [those over eighty-five], loss of muscle strength resulting in frailty is the limiting factor for an individual's chances of living an independent life until death." In study after study, they and others have demonstrated that feebleness in the elderly not only is preventable but, with an appropriate exercise program, can actually be reversed.

In a report now frequently quoted, researchers at Tufts University were able to increase the leg muscle strength of a group of ten frail men and women between the ages of eighty-six and ninety by an average of 174 percent. This was accomplished in a period of eight weeks through a regimen of supervised, high-intensity weight training. Although all of these old folks had chronic diseases or disabilities, none of them sustained any injuries as a result of the exercises. Their balance improved; so did their walking speed. In the nine years since the Tufts group published its results, many confirmatory reports have appeared. Among the surprising findings has been how rapidly the benefits of resistance training with weights become apparent, both by measurements and by improvement in activity.

*   *   *

If you're middle-aged or younger and have read this far, you may be wondering what all of this has to do with you, at least for now. Well, plenty.

Even in our twenties, our ability to manufacture the protein so essential to maintaining muscle begins to lessen. At the same time, fat mass starts to go up and bone density starts to decrease. Though the changes are minimal at first, they speed up after about age thirty, when CT scans actually show evidence of the falling off, such as decreased muscular density and narrower cross-sectional dimensions in the thigh, as well as increasing amounts of fat within individual muscles. Once we reach age fifty, our tendency to dwindle really takes off. Between then and seventy, as much as 30 percent of our strength will be lost, and the process of turning into a little old scarecrow probably doubles in speed. As if all of this were not enough, less muscle and its inevitable result—less activity—mean less stress on the bones, which in turn become less dense and more prone to osteoporosis.

Thus, though loss of muscle strength is the limiting factor for the independence of the oldest old, it quite obviously can have profound effects for the rest of us, too, and much earlier than most people have realized. But cheer up. As the fitness experts tell us, studies that began with the oldest of the old have produced the newest of the news: such deterioration does not necessarily have to take place. The answer, as has only recently been discovered, is anaerobic exercise—activity in which the body incurs an oxygen debt. Aerobics—jogging, running on treadmills, pedaling real or stationary bikes, and the like—may do wonders for the heart and lungs, but to ward off feebleness and its associated debility, nothing replaces resistance training with weights. So impressed has the American College of Sports Medicine been by the demonstrable benefits of resistance exercises that it now recommends weight training for all men and women over the age of fifty.

Weight training has yet another advantage over aerobic exercise: it uses more calories than activities such as walking, running, or swimming. The reason is that heavy exercise breaks down muscle fibers, whose rebuilding by the body's natural reparative processes burns up lots of energy. On top of that, every pound of new muscle requires thirty to forty calories per day just to maintain it, even when it is at complete rest. So it behooves us all, young or old, to hie ourselves to the nearest gym.

Lest you think I am one of those above-it-all types who dish out advice and don't take it, I present here my own personal experience in using the new knowledge. But first I must point out that I did not go gently. For those unconvinced, reluctant, undecided, or indecisive readers— who, in spite of being much impressed with the findings presented in the foregoing paragraphs, are nevertheless shuffling their feet or thinking, "It's all very well and good for you, Mac, but . . . "—well, I will simply say that I have been among your number. But I am now a convert, and like so many converts I am much more than a convert; I am a zealot. Permit me, gentle reader, to explain why I have for nearly a decade been hauling my aging body off to the gym three times a week, there to cavort among the fit.

It all began simply enough. No one—but especially no one as predisposed to vanity as a surgeon—likes to be asked by his eldest son, "Hey, Pops, wouldn't you like to get some tennis shorts that are a little longer, now that your quads aren't what they used to be?" Coming hard on the heels of a longtime tennis partner's across-the-net observation that "our legs are starting to look as if they belong on a couple of scrawny chickens," the thirtysomething's well-intentioned advice was more than a little demoralizing. I decided then and there that the time had come to pay attention to the repeated urgings (truth to tell, they were more like hectorings) of my wife, who had been looking svelter by the day as the result of rising at five each morning to pump iron and run stationary laps at a local gym.

Within days, I had signed up for an exercise program at a facility a few miles from my home called—what else?—the In Shape Fitness Center. Being committed to the principle that all novitiates need a role model, I found myself a deceptively sweet-natured Atlas of a trainer named Dave Butler and told him that I wanted to be just like him when I grew up. Graciously ignoring the obvious fact that I'm thirty-five years older than he, my new mentor took me at my word. Aware that it was far too late to acquire a sweet nature, I nevertheless did harbor an aging male's fantasy about emulating Dave's strength. But first, my immediate goal was to get the old legs back and flatten a gut that was just beginning to make itself evident.

Dave took a long list of measurements, made a series of calculations, and set up a program of resistance training and cardiovascular exercise. It wasn't a menu for the faint of heart, and in spite of his gentle demeanor, Dave proved to be a young man of forceful determination, setting me loose in the gym with the admonition that he expected real improvement by the time I was rechecked in six weeks and then again in eight months.

In matters like these, it helps to have a compulsive personality, and that's where the three-plus decades in the operating room paid off. To this day, I remain religious about my exercise routine, which I labor through at least twice and usually three times a week, always on my own. What do I care that just about every other male in the place is in his twenties or thirties and is pumping as much as twice the iron that I pump? And why be concerned that more than once I have followed a nineteen-year-old coed onto a machine and had to remove twenty or thirty pounds from the weight pile before lifting? The reward came when Dave did that second set of calculations, and even more so at the third.

First, the numbers. In those first eight months of straining, I had taken off nine pounds of fat and added six pounds of muscle mass. My waist was already two inches narrower and my chest an inch and a half wider. The percentage of my body that was fat had dropped from twenty-one (in the range called "acceptable" on the fitness charts) to sixteen (in the middle of the category designated as "fit/healthy"). These improvements came about without an iota's change in my eating habits, although Dave originally outlined a nutrition plan that I to this day gleefully ignore.

And all of this in spite of my traveling schedule. Since I started at the gym, work has often taken me away from home, and there was one period of at least six weeks when I went through the workout no more than a total of four times. Yet I am, in fact, In Shape. I can now run around the tennis court as I haven't since my thirties—or perhaps my twenties. I look forward to my solicitous son's visits, so I can put on (short) bathing trunks, take him to a pool, and show off my (believe it or not) sculpted chest and abdominal muscles, which I have taken to calling pecs and abs. An unexpected dividend has been that almost all of the little muscular aches and pains that we senior citizens force ourselves to get used to began to lessen or even disappear within perhaps a year of beginning my routine.

But there have been a couple of disappointments. It is claimed that consistent strenuous exercise lowers cholesterol. After a small initial drop, mine went right back up to its previous high and has stayed there. Then there's the testosterone story. I'd read reports that its concentration rises with anaerobic exertion, and mine did in fact shoot up to a stratospheric level at the four-month mark, going even higher at a subsequent test. With testosterone like that, I should have been bounding around like a satyr chasing nymphs. When I noticed no change, I queried a friend who specializes in knowing a thing or two about hormones. He gently broke the sad news that heavy exercise increases the secretion of a protein that binds testosterone, which is why its blood level rises. But a bound testosterone molecule is like a bound stallion—it can't run with the herd. It's the *free* testosterone that does the job, and mine has gone up less than 10 percent. But I'm not complaining, and the nymphs are safe.

As for those chicken legs—well, I've never been able to convince my tennis partner to sign up at a gym, but I'm still trying. He's three years older than I, but we both know it's far from too late. And now, so do you.

ACUPUNCTURE IN THE
OPERATING ROOM

Since 1985, I have made a series of journeys to China. Most were undertaken while I was the chairman of the Yale-China Association's medical committee, whose purpose is to oversee a long-standing relationship between the Yale School of Medicine and the Hunan Medical University (recently renamed Xiangya Medical School) in Changsha, a city in south-central China. Like many American physicians, I had become intrigued during that time by what I read of the complex surgical operations being done in the People's Republic with only the use of acupuncture to prevent pain, and I had tried to determine whether such surgery without anesthesia is possible. I had begun my quest in Changsha itself and pursued it in Beijing and Shanghai. What I observed with my own eyes and what I learned through a considerable amount of reading and consultation convinced me that these matters were to be taken seriously.

Before the widespread use of ether as anesthesia after 1846, a number of techniques had been used by surgeons in an attempt to produce some measure of insensibility during operations, the most successful of which involved the ingestion of naturally occurring opiates. Hypnosis, alcohol intoxication, and even a punch in the jaw were well-known methods of inducing stupor but were often either unreliable or unsafe. The introduction of ether and nitrous oxide, and then chloroform in 1847, ended the long search for pain-free surgery; in the last century and a half, and especially in the past fifty years, there has been little need to seek alternative methods. The field of anesthesiology has expanded until it is now one of the most sophisticated of all medical specialties, and this has vastly widened the surgeon's horizons.

But in at least one technologically disadvantaged nation, the search for simpler techniques continued. Until perhaps the past fifteen years, neither the equipment nor the training for contemporary anesthetic methods was easy to come by in the People's Republic of China. The government of the China I used to visit between 1985 and 1991 was besieged by economic, political, and demographic problems to which it appeared to assign higher priority than to the health of individual citizens.

In 1958, Mao Zedong decreed that traditional Chinese medicine be reevaluated in such a way as to incorporate it into the methods of the West, and vice versa. "Make the past serve the present and foreign things serve China," he famously declared. The most dramatic, and best-known, result of this edict was the introduction of the age-old technique of acupuncture into the repertoire of the anesthesiologist. Although acupuncture needles had been used to alleviate pain and symptoms of disease for thousands of years, there is no evidence of their employment in surgery before Mao's dictum.

The acupuncture idea immediately captured the imagination of Westerners, and some were initially prepared to accept the most extravagant success stories that reached their ears. But after the first excitement, conflicting reports of effectiveness began drifting back to the United States and Europe. In the early 1970s, scientists and clinical physicians in various countries organized delegations to visit medical centers in the People's Republic in order to obtain firsthand impressions.

A blue-ribbon study panel of a dozen Americans, sponsored by the National Academy of Sciences in May 1974, was by every criterion the best qualified of the delegations. Its members were expected to provide a definitive response to the charge given them: "To determine how effective this technique is for the prevention or alleviation of pain during surgical procedures." However, after three weeks, during which they visited sixteen hospitals, all that these scientists and clinicians could agree on was that for some patients, under some social and psychological circumstances, undergoing some operations, acupuncture was effective. At best, they suggested, the method might be useful in 10 percent of all surgical cases.

Investigators charged with the intimidating responsibility of verifying a controversial phenomenon like to leave themselves a well-known escape route: they suggest further studies. The brain trust of Americans studying acupuncture was no exception. They recommended that acupuncture anesthesia be further investigated by what they called "well-controlled clinical trials." Although this meant that they had not dismissed the possibility of the technique's usefulness, the average surgeon eagerly awaiting some conclusive word about acupuncture anesthesia was left as much in the dark as before.

I was among those awaiters. On one of my visits, I asked some serious questions of several of the Chinese colleagues I had come to know reasonably well. After returning home, I asked the same questions of a few of the Changsha physicians who were studying at my hospital in New Haven as well as of several Americans who had visited Chinese medical facilities. As my secondhand impressions accumulated, I began to believe that there was a definite role for surgical acupuncture when it was used under very specific conditions. Returning to the academy's report, I saw that it contained data and observations that could support such a conclusion but that the committee, out of either caution or irresolution, had been reluctant to reach it.

I decided to appoint myself a one-man court of inquiry. I was hardly a blue-ribbon panel, for I am neither a scientist nor an anesthesiologist but, rather, an ordinary general surgeon—that is, a surgeon whose operations are limited to the digestive organs, the breast, and the thyroid gland. By that time, however, I did have a comfortable familiarity with a few hospitals in the People's Republic, and, in addition, I had become accustomed to Chinese politeness and the filter of seemingly deliberate obscurity through which everything in that country must be evaluated. I chose to do my personal study in three hospitals in widely separated parts of China, and I sought the help of local surgeons with whom I had previously worked and continued to share long-range interests. I had good reason to believe that they would provide me with an untainted view. I was determined, moreover, to evaluate the accusation of an American urologist friend who warned me one day in an OR locker room, "I know what they do. Somebody told me they slip in a lot of narcotic when you're not looking. The whole thing's a fake."

The first colleague I planned to visit was Dr. Yan Zhangshou, a professor of surgery at the Hunan Medical University with whom I had established a close professional bond on a previous visit. We were men of the same surgical generation and had found plenty of fascinating notes to compare on our first encounter as well as in subsequent letters. When my train pulled into the Changsha railroad station, Yan was waiting on the platform. We didn't try to conceal our pleasure at seeing each other, and there was a great deal to discuss as we slowly drove through the densely crowded streets of the grimy factory city.

When Yan told me that he had asked one of his colleagues to schedule a thyroid operation under acupuncture for the following morning, he made it clear that this was not an unusual performance, since acupuncture was his hospital's preferred anesthetic technique for thyroid surgery. "In some hospitals, the surgeons don't like it," he said. "In the first place, it's not really anesthesia at all. Even people who use that word realize that it doesn't really relieve pain. All it can do is raise the patient's ability to tolerate the pain—his threshold. And for some kinds of pain it doesn't even do a good job of that. We can open a belly with it, but when we begin to pull the intestines around, things become very uncomfortable and the patient always feels nausea—sometimes he vomits. So it's never used for abdominal surgery anymore."

Yan went on to explain that the abdomen is not the only area of the body that presents problems. When a conscious patient is submitted to chest surgery under acupuncture, he must be trained beforehand to control the flow of air into his lungs. Learning to do that takes a lot of instruction, and although many patients can master it, proper breathing under acupuncture is just one more thing for the surgeon and the anesthesiologist to worry about. At the very least, the training delays the operation for a week or more. After some years of variable experience with operations in the chest and abdomen, the method was abandoned as introducing too many risks.

There are two areas of the body where there are no problems of the sort that can be presented by the intestine and the lungs. One of them is the head. In the surgery of brain tumors, Yan told me, acupuncture continued to enjoy some degree of popularity. The other area is the neck, most particularly the lower part of the throat, where the thyroid gland rests its plump, U-shaped fleshiness on the series of cartilage rings that form the skeleton of the larynx, or upper windpipe. The operation I was scheduled to observe was a subtotal thyroidectomy, in which a diseased part of the gland is cut away from the remaining healthy tissue.

When Yan and I arrived at the First Affiliated Hospital of the Hunan Medical University on the following morning, the team of surgeons was just beginning its preparation to remove a two-inch mass from the thyroid gland of Hou Lihui, a thirty-four-year-old woman who worked in one of the many factories of Changsha. When I had written to Yan Zhangshou to tell him that I wanted to see a thyroid operation under acupuncture, her name had been chosen from the list of waiting patients, and she had been admitted a week before I arrived.

During that week, nothing in particular had been done to prepare Mrs. Hou for her operation. She was not visited by the anesthesiologist until the day prior to surgery, and even then her entire period of orientation took less than thirty minutes. Acupuncture is, of course, well known to Chinese patients, even though its use during surgery goes back only fifty years. The anesthesiologist gave her a few suggestions about relaxation and taught her some breathing techniques that might make the procedure less taxing. He promised that she would have only minimal discomfort, or perhaps no discomfort at all.

In the earlier days of surgery under acupuncture, patients were often indoctrinated with the notion that Chairman Mao and the Communist nation would be somehow glorified by each of Chinese medicine's individual victories. Such preoperative political pep talks were abandoned long ago, but in the People's Republic, acupuncture long remained a method of treatment with which patients felt motivated to cooperate fully. Hou Lihui was no exception. She had known of the method since childhood and was as familiar with it as an American is with penicillin shots for strep throat. She had confidence in the hospital, and when the doctors told her she would feel little or no pain during her operation, she took them at their word.

An hour before surgery, a nurse had injected into the muscle of Mrs. Hou's buttock a dose of 40 milligrams of phenobarbital, a barbiturate whose mild action is usually effective for about five hours. As the anesthesiologist, Dr. Xu Qiming, inserted an intravenous line in his patient's left forearm for the infusion of a slow drip of saline solution, he explained to me how he had chosen the acupuncture points he would use. "There are fourteen channels in the body, and we will use two today," he said. "To get a proper result in the front of the neck, we need to make an effect on the liver channel and the stomach channel." These channels, both of which travel across the region of the thyroid gland and are the pathways through which the energy known as *chi* is thought to course, can be accessed at any of a number of points along their extensive length. Different acupuncturists do this in different ways, Xu explained, "but I like the point called Taichong, between the first and second metatarsals, for the liver channel. For the stomach channel, I use Xiangu, between the second and third metatarsals."

Xu sterilized the tops of Mrs. Hou's feet with an iodine solution, and at each of his four chosen points he inserted through her skin a very fine five-inch-long stainless steel needle. He then connected each needle to a small battery to provide what he described as a low-frequency, low-intensity current. "You can buy one of these cheap in a store in downtown Changsha," he said. As the surgical drapes were put in place, Mrs. Hou was given an intravenous dose of 40 milligrams of Demerol and 4 milligrams of droperidol, a tranquilizing sedative that counteracts nausea. Even for a petite woman, these are small to moderate amounts, and they seemed to have little effect on the level of her consciousness. From here on in, the patient herself was generally ignored, except when I directed a question to her through one of the doctors. Her pulse and blood pressure were monitored, and occasional calming words were spoken to her by Xu or his assistant, but otherwise she might just as well have been asleep, sitting partially upright in the standard position for thyroid surgery. A constant stream of conversation was kept up among the staff, much of it the same kind of simple social discourse that is heard in any OR in the world. No attempt was made to generate the cocoonlike atmosphere of quiet reassurance that some theorists believe to be a major factor in the successful application of surgical acupuncture.

Just before making his incision, the surgeon tested the level of pain control, more for my benefit than for his or the patient's—he already knew what the result would be. He picked up a bit of the skin of Mrs. Hou's throat in the serrated tip of a particularly brutal tool called a Kocher clamp and closed the instrument's jaws tightly. Having once or twice had a fingertip snapped up in the vise of a Kocher clamp wielded by an overzealous assistant, I can attest to the agonizing pain it causes, but Mrs. Hou did not so much as flicker an eyelash. Yan smiled broadly as he looked over and saw me shaking my head in disbelief. The patient's lack of response could in no way be attributable to the modest dose of narcotic she had been given; there was clearly some other process at work.

The surgeons worked slowly and meticulously. When the last skin stitch was inserted two and a half hours after the procedure began, Mrs. Hou was just as serene as she had been at the outset. Except for a few fleeting moments of moderate discomfort that she would later describe as a "pinching" sensation, her only complaint had been that maintaining her semiupright position for so long had been difficult. In deference to my New Haven urologist colleague, I had watched the intravenous line carefully, as well as the movements of everyone in the room. Other than the relatively small quantities of barbiturate and narcotic given to the patient before the start of the operation, she had received no drug that could possibly have had any effect on the pain that should have been caused by two and a half hours of surgical excavation in the deep tissues of her neck. Wide awake and smiling at the conclusion of the procedure, she suffered no anesthetic aftereffects. Were it not for the dressing, she would have been indistinguishable from her roommates in the ward, who were awaiting surgery. A few days later, I visited Hou Lihui while making rounds with the surgical team. She had required no postoperative pain medication.

The following week, I saw the same operation done with equal success at the Peking Union Medical College Hospital in Beijing, using different acupuncture points. My guide through that procedure was the retired chief of cardiothoracic surgery, Dr. Xu Letian, who, in the early days of its surgical application, had used acupuncture in all manner of chest operations, including open-heart surgery. Like Yan, he had no certain explanation for the method's effectiveness, or at least none that was yet sufficiently definitive to satisfy a scientifically trained physician unprepared to accept the existence of chi and channels. But as he and I both knew, Chinese and Western researchers have provided some tentative answers to the riddle, and these will be the topic of the next chapter.

CHINESE MEDICINE, WESTERN SCIENCE, AND ACUPUNCTURE

Having witnessed two thyroid operations in which acupuncture successfully substituted for anesthesia, I joined the ranks of the convinced. Though I was certainly *not* convinced of the role said to be played by the mysterious energy called chi or of the existence of channels along which it is said to flow, I had become absolutely sure that the technique was as advertised: it is possible to carry out certain major surgical procedures this way. That I, as a scientifically trained physician, should not only consider such an outlandish possibility but embrace it with enthusiasm might, in the opinion of some, appear to be a wildly erratic departure from the clinical judgment I claim to value so highly.

But there remained the how and the why. I turned first to my surgical colleague Yan Zhangshou, a man reared in the old traditions but trained in the ways of Western science. I am always very careful during conversations in which Chinese therapies are discussed in scientific terms. I'm not sure that such discussions have much validity. Western researchers simply assume that every observable phenomenon must have a straightforward explanation, which they can discover by applying the methods of their kind of science. If no explanation is forthcoming, the scientifically trained mind will usually do one of two things with the unrevealed aspects of the mystery.

The more frequent response is to categorize it as an elaborate, even if not a willful, hoax. Explanations of this sort, which lean heavily on the jargon of the social scientist and the psychologist, are awash with

terms like "autosuggestion," "anecdotal evidence, "cultural expectation," "indoctrination," "selection process," and "uncontrolled." When
the mystery involves sickness, the well-worn "placebo effect" is often
invoked. Many of the Western explainings-away of acupuncture's success, whether in its medical or its surgical uses, have been written in
this kind of language, which effectively begs the question, as do terms
like the ubiquitous "psychophysiological." Invoking such hypotheses
without any evidence except the *lack* of evidence of something more
specific is no elucidation at all, especially when it is the end product of
the very form of Western reasoning that is supposed to abjure fuzzy
thinking.

The second approach is the opposite of the first. In the face of personal observation that cannot be doubted, many a seeker after rational
ways of explaining the as yet unexplainable will try to squeeze it into
one of the pigeonholes of orthodox biomedical science. In the case of
acupuncture, this approach has been theoretical, experimental, or
sometimes both. The theoreticians of acupuncture base their thinking
on a concept called the gate theory, which is that the electricity or the
vast multitude of tiny pain stimuli from the needles so overloads
the capacity of the nervous system that the larger bulk of pain produced by the surgery cannot get to the brain and therefore never en-
ters the patient's awareness. The laboratory scientists have another
idea, and they have produced a host of experimental clues to support it.
Chinese, and some Western, researchers have found evidence that the
stimulation of acupuncture needles often causes the brain to release
narcotic-like substances called endorphins. It is quite possible that
starting up the acupuncture current has much the same effect as starting up an intravenous drip of a powerful drug that acts like morphine.

Even now I have no idea what Yan Zhangshou thinks about all of
this, although I have asked him. He was raised in the certainty of the
Middle Kingdom's superior wisdom, and yet everywhere around him
he sees the urgent demands of the modern science he has been taught.
When he speaks to Westerners—and I am no exception—he seems
obliged to show that he thinks about human biology the way we do, because that is the progressive thing. Yet what can he have done with the
culture he has inherited? Who is he when he is at home?

I like the answer Yan gave me after a long discussion of placebos, the gate theory, and endorphins, because it seems to me that it exemplifies his faith in the possibility that Western science, with its need to believe that it can answer all kinds of eternal questions, may be barking up the wrong tree. Yan's answer was one sentence, deceptively simple. But by his choice of words he managed to communicate his underlying allegiance to the principles of Chinese medicine, his awe of the mysteries of nature, and his willingness to believe that understanding will come. He said, "We don't really know *yet* the natural basis of the channels."

Chinese physicians, despite their upbringing in the old ways, have not been content with explanations based on chi and channels. At the Shanghai Medical University, I visited a research team seeking the scientific basis of acupuncture. My host was the university's president, Dr. Tang Zhaoyou. Tang is a man of my own age, who was for much of his career one of the world's authorities on the diagnosis and treatment of primary liver cancer. His research and surgical contributions are widely known, and his credentials as a clinical scientist are impeccable.

When we discussed my impressions of the thyroid surgery I had seen in Changsha and Beijing, Tang told me of his personal experience as a patient. This was my first opportunity to speak at length with someone who had actually undergone surgery with acupuncture. Even had my own observations left me with significant doubts, any residual skepticism would have been erased by Tang's account, which came, after all, from the director of one of China's leading institutions of Western-style medicine.

"I had thyroidectomy twice under acupuncture," Tang told me. "The first time was in the early 1970s, and it was for benign thyroid tumors. The Cultural Revolution was going on, and things were not so sure. I was a little worried that my recurrent laryngeal nerves might be cut, so I decided that I wanted to talk during the operation, to be safe." (The recurrent laryngeal nerves lie alongside the windpipe on each side of the neck, and they carry impulses to the muscles that move the vocal cords. Because they are situated directly behind the thyroid lobes, they are vulnerable to injury during operation, which inevitably results in permanent hoarseness.) "So I asked for acupuncture, and it went very well. When the condition came back after seventeen years, I needed a total thyroidectomy, to remove all of the remaining gland. I liked acupuncture so much the first time that I had it again. And again, it was fine."

I asked whether he had been given any supplemental sedation. "Only a very small dose of Valium before they started," he replied. "And that second operation lasted four hours."

What did it feel like?

"Well, you know. It's not like complete anesthesia, so I did feel them working—and I could feel touching and pressure. But I had no pain. My real problem was the position. For four hours I had to lie there with my head arched back. That part of it was unpleasant, and made it difficult to swallow my saliva. But otherwise it was good."

What I had heard was a testimonial from a satisfied customer. What impressed me most about the description was the matter-of-fact way in which it was given, as though to say, "Well, of course it was good. What else would you expect?"

Tang arranged for me to meet the director of Shanghai Medical University's Acupuncture Anesthesia and Analgesia Research Coordinating Group, Cao Xiaoding, who in addition to her Chinese medical degree has a doctorate in neurobiology from the Academy of Medical Sciences in Saint Petersburg, Russia. Dr. Cao filled her conversation with talk of experimental protocols, laboratory technology, statistical analysis, and the most fundamental forms of research in neurobiology. In the two hours we spent together, she revealed herself to be a combination of patient pedagogue and incomprehensible fount of abstruse neurophysiological esoterica. I was unprepared to deal with the ultra-sophisticated fruits of her high-powered research team, which consisted of thirty faculty members and six coordinated laboratories of neurophysiology, neuropharmacology, neuromorphology, neurobiochemistry, clinical physiology, and computer science. During an hour of describing experimental studies, Dr. Cao peppered her disquisition increasingly with terms that were only vaguely, if at all, familiar to me, such as "microiontophoretic," "dorsal horn enkephalins," "ventrolateral funiculus," and "radioenzymatic assay." Fortunately, as I was leaving she gave me a gift of journal articles published in English by members of her team, so I was able later to review the vastness of their output while sitting quietly at home surrounded by textbooks and reference materials. What I learned can be summarized in a few paragraphs.

In 1964, the Shanghai researchers began to develop methods to determine the threshold at which pain is felt and the threshold at which it can no longer be tolerated. While studying patients who were undergoing traditional Chinese acupuncture for chronic pain, they and other researchers discovered in the blood an elevation of narcotic-like substances, the so-called endogenous opioid peptides, or endorphins. Later, they were able to demonstrate in animals and in human subjects that these acupuncture-induced endorphins are produced in specific sites in the brain called the caudate nucleus and the periaqueductal gray matter, or PAG. Stimuli applied to those areas increase the amount of endorphin production and also enhance the analgesic, or pain-lessening, effect of acupuncture. Moreover, some American researchers have established that the periaqueductal gray matter contains a relatively high concentration of complex molecular structures called opiate receptors. This means that certain parts of the PAG are the critical sites on which narcotic analgesia has its effect, and those parts are very close to the very cells that produce it. Not surprisingly, when PAG or the caudate nucleus of experimental animals is damaged, the effectiveness of acupuncture is lessened. While traditional Chinese acupuncture is being applied in the usual way, the activity of the two brain centers is increased, and they produce more endorphins. It has been shown that the effect of the increased endorphins, and therefore the effectiveness of the acupuncture, can be partly blocked by the use of nalaxone, a narcotic antagonist. This is supporting evidence that the active agent in acupuncture is indeed the endorphin.

The basic principle described in the Cao group's publications is the same one that has been identified by research teams working in laboratories in America, in Europe, and in other centers in China: acupuncture functions to raise the threshold of tolerance to pain because it activates the body's inherent system of protection. The diminution of pain awareness involves the integrated action of several levels of the nervous system, but the most important factor so far identified seems to be the increased production of endorphins. Of course, the basic question remains: How do the acupuncture needles activate the process in the first place? Dr. Cao's group believes that stimulating the needles sends signals that are picked up by sensory nerves in the area and carried to specific pathways in the spinal cord, which pass them upward to appropriate areas of the brain, including the PAG.

All this provides a reasonable explanation for the effectiveness of surgical acupuncture. But "reasonable" does not mean "proven," nor does it mean even well enough documented to satisfy the rigorous criteria of experimental science. Although there is strong support for Dr. Cao's theories, not all laboratories have been able to replicate her findings, and some legitimate questions have been raised about the experimental methods that were used in her research. Objections like these, however, often arise during the process of validating experimental studies and the theories that develop from them. They are part of the sequence of any scientific inquiry. Whatever the eventual outcome of research in acupuncture, the research itself is certain to increase knowledge about the mechanisms of pain and the body's tolerance of it.

Some Westerners have wondered why it is necessary to await experimental validation before utilizing a technique that has been shown to work in practice. Among them was James Reston, who, until his death in 1995, was one of America's most respected journalists. During his 1971 visit to the People's Republic of China, Reston underwent an appendectomy under spinal anesthesia at the hospital of the Peking Union Medical College. (At that time it had been renamed the Anti-Imperialist Medical College as though in flaunting rejection of the institution's having been founded by that symbol of American hegemony and economic rapacity, the Rockefeller Foundation. When Reston was admitted to the hospital building in which members of the Western diplomatic corps were treated, he saw a large sign just to the right of the entrance, bearing a quotation from Chairman Mao: "The time will not be far off when all the aggressors and their running dogs in the world will be buried. There is certainly no escape for them.")

Much impressed with the acupuncture used to treat his postoperative pain, Reston wanted to learn more. He was taken to operating rooms in a Shanghai hospital where he saw two wide-awake patients undergoing brain surgery with acupuncture. He also saw an alert young man conversing and even eating a piece of fruit while surgeons removed a tuberculous lung through a "vast gaping hole in his back." Of the Chinese surgeons he wrote, "While they cannot agree on the theory of how needle anesthesia works, they are increasingly convinced that it does work, and they are operating on the pragmatic evidence and not waiting for theoretical justifications. . . . There is enough objective evidence of practical medical information in the use of acupuncture to justify exploration by somebody more scientific than newspaper reporters."

Though surgical acupuncture is not being used in the West, many thousands of Americans, perhaps millions, have been treated with its needles for less acute situations, such as chronic pain. One of my colleagues, Dr. Sung Liao, is an expert in this form of therapy. I first met Dr. Liao in 1961. Although our paths have crossed only occasionally during these almost fifty years, it has not been difficult to follow his busy career. A graduate of the Hunan Medical University, he trained in the specialty of rehabilitation medicine at the Massachusetts General Hospital and did further study at St. Thomas's Hospital in London. By the time I caught up with him again, he had founded departments in his specialty in several Connecticut hospitals and was serving as chairman of three of them simultaneously. Until he retired almost twenty years ago, he held the title of clinical professor of surgery at the New York University College of Medicine.

While studying in London, Sung Liao had met Felix Mann, one of England's early proponents of acupuncture, a technique of which Dr. Liao had always been skeptical. "When I was studying at the Hunan Medical University in the 1940s, everything was very scientific," he told me. "We looked down on acupuncture. It was done in the streets." But during the summer of 1971, Dr. Liao suffered the acute onset of rotator cuff syndrome, at which all attempts at nonsurgical therapy failed. In desperation, he sought out Mann, who was at the time lecturing at the downstate branch of the medical school of the State

University of New York. When the condition responded to Mann's acupuncture treatment, Dr. Liao brought together a group of ten physicians to take a course under the master. Gradually, he began to incorporate the technique into the therapy of people who came to him for treatment of a variety of conditions whose major symptom was pain. Once it became known that he was doing this, he was flooded with patients. "When I was at my peak," he told me, "I saw about sixty patients a day. Until 1984, I worked six days a week, usually until ten o'clock at night, and then I gradually cut down to a few hours on two days a week."

Sung Liao estimates that by the time of his retirement he had treated some twenty-five thousand people, with a success rate of about 85 percent, by which he meant no recurrence of pain.

Because doctors, like everyone else, are prone to remember their triumphs more accurately than their defeats, I sought out a disinterested evaluation of Dr. Liao's results. In 1977, Marsha Greenfield, a graduate student at the Yale School of Epidemiology and Public Health, did the research for her master's thesis at Liao's clinic; her dissertation was titled, "Acupuncture as a Rehabilitation Modality in Chronic Low Back Pain Syndrome." Chronic low back pain is a notoriously difficult problem to treat, one that often defies the best efforts of internists, orthopedists, neurosurgeons, and specialists in rehabilitation medicine. Although the underlying pathologies run a wide gamut, all types of low back pain are often lumped together, by physicians and patients alike. People whose pain is resistant to treatment commonly go from one doctor to another until, in desperation, they turn to nonstandard therapies. Many of Dr. Liao's patients had come to him after having undergone manipulation, injection, and even surgery.

Marsha Greenfield studied 220 patients who were treated for low back pain between August 1975 and July 1976. She established specific criteria for improvement and adhered to strict statistical methods in analyzing the results. She found that three-quarters of the patients could be considered to have had a remarkably good response. What makes this figure even more impressive is that so many of them had had histories of therapeutic failure.

Sung Liao is convinced that there are no psychological or personality characteristics that distinguish people who respond to acupuncture from those who do not. He is also convinced—and here he is supported by studies done by others—that there is no relationship between a patient's hypnotizability and the likelihood of response to acupuncture. But like everyone else, he has only theories about why it succeeds so often in chronic cases. Endorphins seem not to play a role, since they have been shown to be elevated only while the needles are in place. Others have disagreed, claiming that breaking the cycle of pain in this way may be the key to its eradication. Still others believe that increased levels of steroids or some other biochemically active substance are the cause, but there is little reliable evidence to support such speculations.

The fact is that the basis of acupuncture's practical usefulness, even in the operating room, has still not been explained in terms acceptable to most orthodox Western scientists using orthodox Western investigative methods. In 1962, Aldous Huxley wrote, in an introduction to Felix Mann's first book, "From telepathy to acupuncture, queer facts get ignored by the very people whose business it is to investigate them—get ignored because they fail to fit into any of the academic pigeonholes and do not suffer themselves to be explained in terms of accredited theories."

But there are philosophers of science and medicine who tell us that we are on the threshold of a new way of looking at and interpreting the observations we make of the processes of disease and health. The effectiveness of correctly applied acupuncture is not our only evidence that there are undeniable phenomena that cannot—at least not yet, as Yan Zhangshou would put it—be explained by the investigational methods of today's biomedical science. Other functions may be involved, and perhaps philosophies may be required beyond those that have been so successful since the scientific method became a major current of Western thought. Maybe the new perspectives will have room for such concepts as yin, yang, chi, and channels. Maybe they will not. Either way, I find myself agreeing with James Reston: we should get on with it.

THE MISTY CRYSTAL BALL

While watching the huge ball drop at midnight on New Year's Eve 2000, I realized that I, too, had dropped the ball. For months, I had been pontificating to anyone who sought medical predictions for the coming century, sparing few of my inquirers the verbal vanity of an opinionated man who spends too much time alone, scribbling in a small room. Yet in a series of musings dedicated to the uncertainty of the art of healing, I had written not a word about the next hundred years. What, in fact, could be more uncertain than the future of medicine?

I suppose there may have been someone who, in 1800, foresaw the germ theory and the transformation it would wreak on medical thought; or the notion that the origin of disease should be sought in cells rather than in the affected organs themselves; or perhaps the revolution in surgery that would make possible the removal of entire lengths of the digestive tract without destroying the quality of life.

And I suppose also that there may have been someone who, in 1900, foresaw the invention of machines that would allow the inside of a stilled heart to be surgically invaded and its valves repaired; or the commonplace transplantation of organs; or, *mirabile dictu*, the era of molecular biology that is causing medical thought to be transformed once again, even more than it was transformed by germ theory in the nineteenth century.

But if such Nostradamuses did exist, there is no written evidence. Viewed retrospectively, what might appear to be leaps achievable only with the scientific equivalent of seven-league boots can be recognized in each case to have been the result of a long series of small achievements, many of which are now forgotten by all but a few specialized historians of medicine. Those who did the prevenient work rarely had any idea what their studies and experiments were leading to; the research was done for its own sake or with short-term goals in mind, and not, until the transforming discoveries came into view, as part of some long-range plan that might have been predicted by knowledgeable seers at the beginning of a century.

Now, as before, there are researchers who, in the words of Longfellow, are slowly "toiling upward in the night," having no idea how their increments of work will shift the currents of biomedical science. Or perhaps some of them do have an idea, but it is likely to be wrong. What is thought to lead down a specific avenue often takes another direction, and successive discoverers find themselves on a hitherto unforeseeable journey. It was only in the century just passed that the growth of science began to be subjected to the scrutiny of philosophers and historians, and they have taught the rest of us about the undirected ways in which knowledge really does evolve.

The result is that there is nowadays a much greater appreciation of the complexities of scientific discovery than there was one or two hundred years ago, and this should help us recognize the hazards of attempting to foretell progress beyond the next decade or so. But some of us stubbornly refuse to learn from the lessons of the past two centuries; we are not fazed by the unfulfilled forecasts of our predecessors. We would-be prophets cannot resist plunging into the predictive waters, though with varying degrees of recklessness. Being more aquatically (and oracularly) timid than most, I'll restrict myself here to sticking a toe in—or perhaps I'll wade out just a bit, but not far enough to get in over my head. After all, putting prophecies into print is quite different from simply mouthing off about them.

In the spirit of toe sticking, I'll start with one of the innovations that is already beginning to come into view, by which I mean that it will be affecting a significant number of patients by the second decade of this century. It doesn't seem risky to foresee the almost visible dawn of the day when pharmacologic agents will be tailored to the genetic characteristics of specific diseases and even specific patients. As the genetic contribution to more and more pathologies is identified, it will become increasingly possible to engineer drugs for individuals that will correct or head off abnormalities. Gene therapy is still far from living up to the hopeful assertion made in 1996 by the founder of the field, W. French Anderson: "Twenty years from now, gene therapy will have revolutionized the practice of medicine. Virtually every disease will have gene therapy as one of its treatments." But the hour is still early. Though there is no general agreement that the boldness of Anderson's statement is justified, at least this aspect of it—the engineering of patient-specific drugs—appears to be coming ever closer to realization. And the rest of its implications cannot be ignored either. In spite of failures and at least one tragedy, no sensible biomedical scientist is giving up on the scenario that Anderson continues to believe is realistic, though most do question his notion of the time required to achieve it. Even the much heralded replacement (or perhaps repair) of disease-related genes may not be as far off as some pessimists think, notwithstanding its present chaotic state of development.

Another innovation that can be anticipated—one even closer in many ways than genetically based drugs—is the imminent revolution in diagnostic imaging. The various types of scanning now available, and most particularly the rapidly improving technology of what is called functional magnetic resonance imaging (fMRI), which allows the study of chemical reactions, will soon provide opportunities for investigating disease processes in ways that will make current X-ray techniques and other radiologic methods seem absurdly simplistic. It is not too farfetched to look forward to the day (which will probably come before midcentury) when biopsies, blood tests and other tissue and fluid samples, exploratory surgery, electrocardiograms, and similar studies of function and structure will be obsolete. Technicians will place patients in scanning chambers in which all manner of pictures will be produced to elucidate bodily mechanisms, right down to the level of intracellular activities. The pinpointing of many of the factors that contribute to the complexities of disease will be enormously enhanced—at, of course, an unavoidably enormous expense.

Not only clinical medicine but basic research, too, will benefit from the new technology, because imaging will contribute to the other modalities that explain the molecular origins of disease. More understanding will bring less need for the draconian measures that currently constitute our surgical corrections of pathology. As biochemical and genetic therapies replace surgery, the therapeutic approach to many diseases will undergo vast changes. Surgical treatment of cancer will be the first to diminish and then disappear, followed in succeeding decades by the operative treatment of cardiovascular, congenital, and inflammatory diseases. By the end of the century, the operating room will be essentially a place to treat trauma and insert newly crafted parts. John Hunter, the eighteenth-century Scotsman who introduced his fellow surgeons to the methods of science, once remarked that operations are a barbarian's method of achieving ends that wiser men would reach by strategy. During the course of the twenty-first century, we will become biomedically much wiser than we are today.

But until that wisdom has fully evolved, it will be necessary to bring the ancient craft of surgery closer to the present technological era, and that will take place within the next two decades. Here, too, imaging will play an important role. The combination of increasingly sophisticated CT scanning and MRI will show us an accurate three-dimensional representation of diseased anatomical structures. After a patient has been anesthetized, slender externally wired instruments will be inserted into the body through tiny incisions: laser-based tissue vaporizers to replace present-day scalpels and scissors, welding devices to replace stitches and staples. The surgeon will sit at a console before two screens, one showing the area to be operated upon and the other a simulation of the proposed operation. Using a sort of navigation system, he will superimpose the operation on the anatomy and then program the entire procedure to be carried out by the instruments. Not only will the system be voice-operated, but the surgeon may even have several consoles in front of him, so that as many as six operations can be done at once. Because the probes will be inserted and connected to their electronic directing source by technicians, the surgeon will be able to do all his work from a remote location—even from the other side of the world. Aftercare beyond the first few days will be overseen via a monitoring device placed in the patient's home, so that no postoperative visits will be needed. Some operations for trauma may even be performed at the scene of injury, which will greatly decrease the accident and battlefield mortality rate. Soldiers will carry small monitors into combat, enabling them to be located immediately upon being wounded so that corpsmen may do the initial first aid and insert probes.

Research with stem cells, those primordial units of life with the potential to develop into any of the body's constituent tissues, will change the face of medical therapy, especially that which deals with congenital defects and with the effects of such degenerative diseases as arteriosclerosis and arthritis. Transplantation may very well become obsolete by midcentury, as the bioengineers partner themselves with the stem cell pioneers to create new organs crafted by combining designer cells with mechanical devices. The new field called biomimetics has already given us artificial joints, heart valves, intraocular lenses, and the like, but these kinds of structures are only the first of many possibilities likely to spring from the union of the two disciplines.

We constantly hear about the "Century of the Brain," but that era has long since begun and will long continue, overlapping any temporal borders. Studies of the nature of consciousness and of the relationships between brain and mind and between mind and body will bring insights that have been sought since ancient times. Developments in these areas will reveal the mechanisms by which nonscientific approaches to healing, such as those we call traditional medicine, can be effective under appropriate circumstances. The real mechanism by which factors such as faith, psychological profile, suggestion, and placebos sometimes influence outcome will be critically scrutinized. The vast amount of chaff will be separated from the priceless wheat, and orthodox medicine will incorporate the results into the armamentarium of scientifically based healing.

The laboratory theorists will continue to raise the specter of increasing the human life span to unjustifiable, if not frankly dangerous, lengths. But common sense will prevail, and the research in aging that is of real value will be devoted to the improvement of the added years of life we have already been given and the few more that the other advances will provide. Attention will be focused on the notion of what has been called "compression of morbidity," by which is meant the conversion of the present slow decline in the health of the aged to a pattern in which vitality is maintained until shortly before death.

Of those advances that can be predicted, the most flabbergasting will be the creation of life in the laboratory. Whatever may be the real nature of life as defined by theologians, philosophers, and poets, its strictly physiological characteristics can be found in any textbook of elementary biology. To qualify, organic material must grow, respond to stimuli, digest, reproduce, and fulfill several other functions. This requires at least the minimal set of genes that permit these functions to be carried out. Scientists are still a long way from identifying what this so-called minimal genome might consist of, but they are hard at work trying to find out. Because it is already possible to build small segments of DNA, it makes sense that such a genome might be synthesized once its constituent structures are known. A project like this takes the insights of many thousands of researchers and can proceed only by small increments over a long time. But there seems little question that such a thing will come about by the year 2100. It is not impossible that an entire organism, even a multicellular one, may be created in the laboratory by then. The implications for medicine of such an achievement are huge, but the first of them will be the opportunity to study the ways in which life processes go awry to cause disease. And there will be also be therapeutic possibilities, such as the use of synthesized organisms in the fight against pathogens and genetic abnormalities.

All of these predictions are well within the bounds of reason. The probabilities of their fulfillment are so high, in fact, that no Wizard of Odds would dare bet against them. What cannot, of course, be known is the nature of the unforeseeable series of events that will once again transform medical thinking. Although the fact that each of the last five centuries has witnessed a transforming upheaval in medicine does not necessarily mean that it is likely to happen again, I hereby (at the risk of leading you astray, trusting reader) express my confidence that it will. I do recognize the hazards of listening to people like me, whose baleful effect on others was pointed out more than three hundred years ago by Blaise Pascal in his *Pensées:* "All the misfortunes of men arise from one single thing, which is their inability to sit still in a small room at home." But even so, I stick by my forecast that something enormous will take place that is at present unpredictable. Should the future prove me to have been only a troublemaking false prophet, my critics will by then have to organize a séance in order to tell me so.

The foregoing are medical or scientific predictions. But there will be yet another innovation that fits into neither of those categories, and it will result in consequences as profound as any of those already enumerated. I refer to the change that will appear in society's attitude toward its own involvement in biomedicine. First, priorities in the application of new discoveries and, then, priorities in research will within a few decades be determined by a consensus of the public and scientific communities. This will come about as a result of society's increasing realization that the moral and ethical implications of the new biomedicine demand the attention of all of us. Though scientists currently resist this sort of societal input, they will come to an appreciation of its importance as they make decisions that reflect their obligation to vouchsafe the future of our species and its environment. This new partnership will refuse to let the present unsatisfactory state of science education in this country persist. And this brings me to my final prediction: if for no other reason than the sheer necessity of increased involvement, we will see vast changes in the educational system, with great improvements in the average American's knowledge of science.

Each of the past four centuries has seen an exponential increase in the number of people doing science and an exponential increase in the complexity of the enterprise. The breathtaking achievements of the researchers have been made at the cost of great individual dedication and sacrifice, and in more than a few instances at the cost of researchers' lives, whether directly or indirectly. Basic scientists are men and women apart, and the rest of us who benefit from their contributions do so without very often stopping to think of the price that many of them have paid and continue to pay in terms of personal well-being. We take for granted that every generation will produce young people so fascinated by the study of nature that they will forgo more readily attainable pleasures—and financial remunerations—to pursue this particular form of truth. We have even become glib—as have I in this essay—about our expectations of what they should provide for us.

There is a greatness about many of these people, and a patience and persistence that dwarfs the endurance of all but a few dedicated strivers in other fields. They are the ones about whom Longfellow might have been thinking when he wrote the line quoted in the first part of this essay. Here is the entire passage in which his words appear, from "The Ladder of Saint Augustine":

> The heights by great men reached and kept
> Were not attained by sudden flight,
> But they, while their companions slept,
> Were toiling upward in the night.

HIDDEN MEANINGS

The notion of sympathy among various organs of the body has existed since ancient times. As recently as 150 years ago, in fact, it was still a major influence on medical thought. Physicians theorized that events and qualities—even moods—originated in one structure and affected the behavior of others, usually the ones closest to it. Of course, we now know that something of this sort does indeed take place, not only through the nervous system, but also through blood-borne messengers like hormones.

Yet the kind of sympathy believed in by the ancients and near moderns was something quite different from the nerve- or hormone-induced physical and chemical activities we study today. In that long-ago era, when emotions were thought to originate in various organs (particularly the heart, stomach, liver, and spleen), certain parts of the body were said to commune with one another. The Romans, for example, placed the origin of moodiness and wrath in the stomach and claimed that these feelings appear only secondarily in the heart. At a time when many were convinced that the heart was the seat of the mind, it is not surprising that passions and thoughts were believed to be transmitted between the stomach and the heart by means of the vaguely defined "sympathy" that they shared.

If this is true, reasoned the theorists, then any structure lying between these two major organs must also be imbued with the characteristics that pass from one to the other. Based on this kind of construction, the Greek *phrenes*, the transverse sheet of muscle we call the diaphragm, became the origin of *phren*, meaning "the mind" or "the seat of the emotions." From those beginnings arose *frenetic, schizophrenic,* and *phrenology*, the name of the pseudoscience that purports to diagnose mental and psychological states from the assessment of skull contours.

In such ways does our language reflect the history of medicine and our attempts to understand our bodies and their relation to the cosmos.

Perhaps the richest source of the language that originates in conceptions about our own inner workings is the theory of humors. There are Greek texts dating from approximately 500 B.C.E. that describe the dependence of the body's physical and emotional harmony on the balance of four fluids, or humors: blood, phlegm, yellow bile, and black bile. When the four exist in proper equilibrium, according to the theory, all is well and the individual is healthy and serene. But should one or another of them become either excessive or diminished, sickness ensues, its precise form depending on the nature of the imbalance. Therapy is directed toward restoring the original state of stability.

Blood, for example, warmed by an innate heat supposedly generated in the heart, was said to quicken the spirit. When an illness was characterized by elevated body temperature, flushing, agitation, or perhaps a fast pulse, it was treated by removing some of the excess blood. Such measures as purging, blistering, sweating, emetics, and enemas were employed to rid the body of other imbalances, either by forcing certain humors out of it or by bringing them to the surface. These practices formed the basis of standard therapies until well into the nineteenth century, and continued long afterward in the treatment schemes advocated by grandmothers and other such sages of kitchen wisdom. Mustard plasters, cupping, high colonics, and the steam room have a long history in the annals of healing.

According to the original Greek system, it was not only sickness and health that were influenced by the humors. One's personality was affected—to a great extent determined—by the particular baseline combination of the four fluids that was unique to each individual. Since each humor imparted its own characteristics, a person's behavior was a reflection of the way in which the humors were mixed together. As the centuries passed, certain qualities of personality came to be known by the Greek or Latin names of the humors thought to be their basis.

Thus, if someone was lively, ardent, or optimistic—sanguine, in a word—it was because his dominant humor was blood, for which the Latin is *sanguis*. For reasons shrouded in mystery, yellow bile came to be associated with anger or discontent, resulting in the origin of our word *choleric*, from the Greek *chole*, or "bile." When someone is bilious, he can thank the Latin *bilis* for that designation, unless he is so confrontational that he has too much gall to thank anyone for anything. As for *phlegmatic*—it speaks for itself, especially when one considers that phlegm was thought to come from the brain. There is a bit of paradox here, or at least an inconsistency, because the loss of phlegm (meaning the loss of brain) rather than its excess was believed to be the reason that some people become dull and sluggish, or perhaps just imperturbable.

Black bile has a story all its own. The other three humors are easily visible under appropriate circumstances, but black bile was an enigma. It had been added to the other three in order to achieve some symmetry in a formulation that might be called "the notion of fours." This thesis had been brought forth by the fifth-century-B.C.E. philosopher Empedocles, who declared that everything in the universe is made up of varying combinations of air, earth, fire, and water. If this is so, and if there are four seasons, the number of humors must also be four—but what to do with the fact that only three were readily identifiable? The solution, in more ways than one, was to invent a fourth. No one knows who hit on the idea of black bile, but it sounds like the kind of thing dreamed up by a committee. Subsequent generations tried to prove its existence by pointing to what they considered visible evidence, like the blackish exudations that sometimes ooze from tumors and sick organs, but such arguments were recognized as weak, if not patently specious. The fact is that there is no such thing as black bile, though no Greek-influenced thinker would ever admit it.

Having brought it into the world despite its imaginary nature, the ever-resourceful doctors and philosophers had to associate the mythical humor with an organ. If the heart had its blood, the liver its yellow bile, and the brain its phlegm, what structure could possibly be the best domicile for black bile? The answer, as obvious as it was, seemed too good to be true. Tucked up under the left side of the rib cage was a fist-shaped, dark-hued collection of flesh whose function no one had ever been able to fathom. Though the Greeks and preceding civilizations had assigned a job to virtually every other viscus, the spleen was without identifiable employment. Perhaps in desperation, Aristotle called it "a bastard liver," but others disagreed. In the second century c.e., Galen would come to refer to it as *plenum mysterii organum*, "the organ full of mystery," and suggest fanciful roles for it in the general economy of the body.

Being without any other certain function and deep purplish red in color—becoming much darker the moment blood stopped flowing through it—the spleen seemed the perfect location for the origin of black bile. The organ's funereal color contributed verisimilitude to its humor's fictional role, the formation of disposition and personality: a surfeit of black bile was the cause of melancholy. In fact, the very word comes directly from the Greek theories of human biology. Since *melas* is "black," barely a short skip reaches the derivation of "melancholy" from *melas* and *chole*.

The association of melancholy with the spleen had great appeal to people of succeeding eras. The word "spleen" eventually became the name of a disease, which, judging by its characteristics as described in medical and lay literature of the seventeenth and eighteenth centuries, was identical to the spectrum of symptoms we nowadays call depression. But something had been added along the way. Perhaps because of an intuitive recognition of the psychological relationship between depression and repressed anger, the expression "to have an attack of the spleen" was often used to mean that the person in question was angry or discontented—in other words, splenetic. The best way to avoid overt manifestations of such a state of mind was to "vent one's spleen," which in essence meant opening up the organ to allow escape of the accumulated black bile.

Black bile is the most storied of the humors, but blood, long recognized as the carrier of the vital energy, is the most dramatic. One of the earliest interpretations of physiology—one that must have been made even by the thinking predecessors of Homo sapiens—was that blood carries the life-giving force. An injury resulting in considerable loss of blood was seen to leave its victim seriously weakened; if enough of the rich red fluid exited the body, life itself went with it. To the first healers, the huge spongy liver appeared to be choked with blood and was therefore believed to be the site where blood was manufactured. If this were so, the liver must indeed be the seat of life, a notion that would find linguistic expression in the Indo-European root *leip*, a term associated also with the concept of being alive. It is from this source that the word "liver" originates, as does the word "life" itself. In German, the organ is called *die Leber*, and the verb "to live" is *leben*. Our language has inherited the ancient notion that the liver is the organ that makes it possible for us to live.

Of all the words that ancient medical theory has contributed to the vocabulary of modern English, there is none whose original meaning— or at least a close approximation—persisted as long as "hysteria." Its origin is to be found in the uterus, for which the Greek word was *hystera*. Civilizations long before theirs had attributed magical powers to the reproductive organs, but the *hystera*, concealed deep within the female pelvis, had a lore all its own. It was said to roam throughout the body, unrestricted by such natural boundaries as the diaphragm or the upper rim of the chest. It might lodge like a globular obstruction in the throat, a condition that in time came to be called *globus hystericus*; when feeling acutely overheated, it leaped toward the abdominal wall, hoping to be cooled by the outside air; if the problem was thirst, it would throw itself forcefully at the liver in order to be moistened by the nearby humors. Leaping and plunging were not its only means of locomotion: sometimes the uterus would meander in a leisurely fashion around the inside of a woman's body, seeking, seeking—who knows what it was seeking, or why?

Plato thought he had the answer. In *Timaeus*, he asserted that the organ acted out of frustration with its unfulfilled desire to nurture new life. Calling it "an animal within an animal," he proclaimed as certainty a theory already accepted by many earlier students of the subject: "When it remains unfertilized for a long time during the proper season the uterus becomes seriously angry and moves all over the body." Others claimed that the frustration arose from a cause prior to fertilization. It was the sexual act itself, they declared, and all of the pleasures attendant on it that were missing from the life of the *hystera*. The set of symptoms caused by uterine peregrinations became known as hysteria, and they were assumed to have a sexual cause.

Those symptoms covered a wide range, attributable to the erratic movements of the uterus. A woman's otherwise unexplainable abdominal pain, choking, shortness of breath, fainting, heartburn, headache—all these were due to hysteria, according to the physicians of the classical period, the Middle Ages, the Renaissance, and beyond, almost to our own time. As late as 1979 the *Diagnostic and Statistical Manual of the American Psychiatric Association* still listed "Hysterical Neurosis" as a disease. In the association's defense, it must be said that precious few psychiatrists seem to have had any idea of the origin of the term. We are thus confronted with the ludicrous spectacle of an entire learned profession pleading ignorance to avoid blame.

There seems little doubt that some symptoms now placed within the broad category of "psychosomatic," or perhaps designated by the far more restricted term "conversion reaction," can in certain cases be traced to sexual conflicts. This is a far cry from the assurance with which physicians of earlier eras viewed the disease they called hysteria. They did not hesitate to base their therapies on the millennia-old conception, as it were. If a patient was married, they prescribed pregnancy; if not, she was to be sexually satisfied by clinical means. Until the turn of the twentieth century, manual doctor-induced orgasm was an accepted therapy. The vibrator, in fact, was invented in the 1880s with this very clinical purpose in mind. Those who view with nostalgia that earlier time before instruments replaced the doctor's touch might look on such an innovation as a mixed blessing.

The induction of pregnancy and orgasm were treatments of the kind that a modern physician would call "interventional." But simpler means were sometimes used to achieve much the same objective, while avoiding the laying on of hands. Being an animal, reasoned the ancients, the uterus should be attracted by pleasant smells and repelled by noxious ones. All manner of concocted vapors were inhaled through the nose or wafted up into the vagina to induce the smell-sensitive organ to move down into the pelvis. Ambroise Paré, the renowned sixteenth-century French surgeon, recommended "sweet and aromaticke fumigations" emanating from a long-necked metal vessel under which a fire was lit. A detailed drawing in his widely read textbook, translated into English in 1634, depicts the vessel, fire and all, positioned between a standing woman's widespread legs. Fumes flow upward from a mixture of cinnamon, lavender, benzoin, pennyroyal, calamine, nutmeg, musk, "and such like, which for their sweet smell and sympathy, allure or entice the wombe downewards."

The male reproductive organs, too, are not without their contribution to etymology. The flower we call an orchid derives its name from its ball-shaped double root, the sight of which brings to mind the Greek word *orchis*, meaning "like a testicle." When a man is in a hospital awaiting orchiectomy, he is not about to have flowers removed from his room. Rather, he is scheduled for excision of his testicles, a procedure formerly used to diminish hormone secretion in certain cases of prostate cancer.

Some men would rather lose their souls than their testicles. In earliest times and in societies we call primitive, the loss of the soul, followed by its immediate retrieval, was thought to be a common occurrence. The underlying philosophy that made such an event possible was the notion that humans, being part of the cosmos, are made of the same materials as everything else in the universe. To the Greeks, these were the aforementioned air, earth, fire, and water. In their formulation, the entire cosmos is motivated and energized by a poorly defined power that is variously called soul, spirit, pneuma, psyche, anima (there are small differences in the meaning and usage of these words, but for our present purposes they are interchangeable), and several other names, depending on the culture. Being a microcosm of the macrocosm, each of us derives our soul from the soul of all that surrounds us in the universe—we bring it inside ourselves by the act of breathing. *Psyche*, or *psuche*, in fact, Greek for "soul" or "spirit," is derived from an Indo-European root that refers to breathing. Throughout history, a sneeze has been thought to propel the soul out of the body. Though we think of this concept as a superstition nowadays, it had the blessing (in

more ways than one) of orthodox philosophy in Greek-influenced societies. The best way to get the soul back was to utter some slogan that
was essentially a prayer. And from this comes "Gesundheit" and "God
bless you." These ancient confabulations die hard. Try leaving the
proper formula unspoken the next time a friend sneezes, and note how
the anxiety level rises until the magical saying has been uttered.

So God bless you all, and Gesundheit. This talky tale is done, along
with whatever lesson may be found in it. Alas, the day when an abundance of philologists graced the faculties of major universities is long
past. The history of our culture is hidden in the unexamined history of
our words, and there it will remain. We let them fly from our lips heed-
lessly, without a moment's wonder.

IS THERE A DOCTOR IN THE HOUSE?

Al Capp invented a host of colorful minor characters for his acclaimed comic strip, "Li'l Abner." Whenever there is a cardiac emergency in a public place, I feel like one of them: a lugubrious little fellow over whose head a small black cloud always hovered. His name was Joe Bfstplk, the surname meant to be pronounced like a Bronx cheer. The cloud connoted disaster, and disaster was precisely what Joe brought with him everywhere he went.

My own little black cloud is heart-shaped. It has made its ominous appearance in theaters and concert halls, during transatlantic flights (note the use of the plural in each case, which should not necessarily be taken to mean merely two), and on the street. While still newly graduated, I used to think that the sentence "Is there a doctor in the house?" was the intro to some hilarious sequence in a Marx Brothers movie or a vaudeville routine. I soon learned otherwise. Some people actually do use that formula when a physician is needed in a hurry. Those are precisely the words that have ushered in some of the most memorable episodes of my life. More often than not, they have ended badly.

My first such experience seems to have presaged the future. The date was November 1961, and the occasion was the first night out together that my wife and I had spent since the birth of our daughter six weeks earlier. I had completed my specialty training at the beginning of the summer and was working hard at my new job, which was to initiate a program of open-heart surgery at a midsized hospital in New York. I was earning the munificent sum of twelve thousand dollars a year, a fourfold increase over the salary I had been paid during the sixth and final year of my residency at the Yale–New Haven Hospital.

Feeling flush with such unaccustomed wealth and vaulted into an expansive mood by the nature of the occasion we were celebrating, I had splurged by buying two center-section aisle seats in the tenth row of the Booth Theatre, where Julie Harris was starring in a critically hailed production of *A Shot in the Dark*. The general feeling of well-being—and financial abundance—expanded to include a romantic pretheater dinner at an intimate café nearby, so that by the time my wife and I arrived fifteen minutes before the performance, both of us were at peace with the world and prepared to let the thespian magic of Miss Harris and her company of actors wash over us for the next two hours.

We settled into our seats, smiled beneficently at the couple along-side us, perused the program with the insouciance of two young so-phisticates long accustomed to frequenting this purse-favored part of the theater, and prepared for the curtain to go up. We were feeling comfortable in every sense of the word.

All at once, the subdued conversational hubbub and bustle of that quintessential Friday-evening theater audience was pierced by the sound of a man yelling out an unintelligible sentence in a high-pitched, fretful voice. He reached the final syllable just as the pre-curtain buzz began to respond to the alarming intrusion by quickly dying down, as each of us in that vast room became quiet, straining to hear the words being shouted. The result of his momentary halt, and ours, was a deep-ening hush, finally so complete that the auditorium was filled with an intense silence. The aura of stillness had an eerie quality, as if, with one pair of ears, we were awaiting a sound that we had been forewarned would break a spell. The wait lasted barely a moment before the expec-tant emptiness of air was suddenly filled with the urgent blast of "Is there a doctor in the house?" Now that I heard it clearly, I recognized that my disbelieving mind had actually understood those words the first time they entered it. Even through the babble of voices, I had known what was being said. But it seemed to make no sense.

People don't actually talk that way in real life—I was sure of that. Bursting out with such a hackneyed phrase had to be someone's idea of a practical joke, or perhaps it was the raving of a deranged man. The only problem with my thesis was that the second outcry had apparently paralyzed the members of the audience into an utter absence of motion. They were taking the loud summons seriously. All around me, men and women sat stiffly in their seats, and a few looked as though they had actually shrunk down into the plush in an attempt to hide from being called upon to do something. With all onlookers frozen this way, my vista was clear. I could now see that the source of the commotion was a uniformed usher, standing alongside an elderly man slumped onto the arm of his aisle seat in the front row of the side section.

I leaped up and bounded toward the stricken man. He was unresponsive, pulseless, and blue. His equally elderly seatmate, who I later learned was his sister, was hysterical. When I told her I was a doctor, she began to scream into my ear that he had a heart condition, as if that message itself would confer magical powers on me if repeated again and again, or perhaps would bring her brother back from what was an obvious cardiac arrest.

The treatment for cardiac arrest is external massage, with or without intermittent propulsion of air into the windpipe. In 1961 it was thought to require two people, one to compress the breastbone and the other to force breath into the victim's mouth. It had not yet been realized that both could be done by one person, alternating the two maneuvers in appropriate sequence: cardiopulmonary resuscitation. I seized my patient by the shoulders and threw him to the carpeted floor alongside the row. The sight was too much for his sister. Sobbing violently, she rushed toward the exit.

On my knees and straddling that inert body in the center of the aisle, I began a rhythmic series of compressions on the lower part of my suddenly acquired patient's sternum. As I completed the first series of thrusts, I looked up at the audience members near me, assuming that someone would come forth to do the mouth-to-mouth breathing. The astonishing sight that greeted my eyes was one not easily forgotten.

Despite the tumult that had initiated it, no one in that entire capacious place seemed prepared to admit awareness of the drama being played out within a few feet of the stage. Even when I momentarily lifted my crouching body to survey the auditorium and what was visible of the balcony, I saw not a single face, except my wife's, turned in my direction. In order not to be confronted with the obvious, each of the other audience members had suddenly discovered something to become fascinated by, something that required unwavering attention. The chandeliers were particularly popular, but the cynosure of many other eyes was one or another portion of the curtain. Some stared fixedly at a red EXIT sign; others focused intently on their programs, as though trying to memorize each printed word. These people would under no circumstances allow themselves to be distracted from their determined dissociation. I was being studiously ignored. The panicky usher had disappeared, and I was left alone in that sea of inaccessible theatergoers with only the unconscious man for company and my wife's tight-lipped imitation of a smile for encouragement.

But I was not alone for long. Perhaps the tension was proving too much for a fortyish fellow in the middle of the twelfth row. Whatever the reason, he suddenly—but not until three or four minutes had passed—pulled himself up from his seat and began clambering toward me over the unmoving legs of his neighbors, finally tripping on the inert ankles of the stolid occupant of the aisle seat, who kept staring straight ahead, trying to appear unaware of anything going on around him. On reaching my side, the new volunteer asked me, in a soft middle European accent, what to do, and I told him. Without hesitating, he applied his lips tightly to those of our moribund companion, and began to blow air forcefully into his gaping mouth while squeezing shut the man's two cyanotic nostrils with his fingertips.

We continued our efforts for about ten more minutes, though I had known almost from the start that the old man's life was beyond retrieval. But he had one more trump in him: with a single great spasm of his terminally twitching abdominal muscles—it must have been timed in perfect synchrony with an agonal contraction of his stomach—he vomited directly into the mouth of his would-be rescuer. Thus did our patient let us know that he was dead, and it was time to stop.

I got up from straddling the corpse, my dismay at the outcome of the situation somewhat lessened by its manifest inevitability. I thanked my partner and shook his hand, then surveyed the audience again. Even now that it was safe, no one so much as glanced at us. We stood alone in that small dark circle of death, surrounded by a vast penumbra of indifference. Whatever had been found so alluring about the curtain, the chandeliers, and the EXIT signs had lost not a bit of its attraction. Hundreds of avid eyes were still glued to programs, though some of them were growing a bit glassy. Half a dozen policemen were bustling their way down the aisle toward us, no doubt summoned by the disappearing usher or one of his colleagues. It was then that I realized that no member of the theater's staff had appeared on the scene. After exchanging a few words with the cops, my partner and I repaired to the men's room. He rinsed his mouth over and over. We returned to our seats as unregarded as when we had left them.

A few of the theater's management people finally made an appearance. The police asked them some questions and then lifted the body off the floor to carry it out. I couldn't resist standing up to see whether even this final moment in the lethal drama would be diligently ignored by the audience. It was. A few of the curtain starers had no doubt switched over to reading their programs, or an EXIT sign aficionado may have turned his face up to a chandelier, but otherwise everything was just as it had been at the beginning. In that place of stony quiet, the humanity of three people had been dismissed. Throughout the entire episode, we had been more than ignored—we had been forcefully extruded from everyone's consciousness. Not until the cops and the corpse were out of the auditorium did the usual theater hubbub start up again, as though the intervening thirty minutes had not happened. The audience sat back after a bit, the curtain went up, and the show began—or at least the show that everyone had come to see.

That episode of group avoidance took place on a Friday evening at a Broadway theater. Who knows how many physicians were in the audience—ten, twenty, far more? Some of them must even have been seated within yards of the dying man, but no one came to his aid. They behaved like everyone else in that place, determined not to become involved and in their case evading implicit responsibility. It was my first experience with this phenomenon, but hardly my last. I would see it several times more over the years, but I would more frequently see its opposite. I once attended a concert in New Haven where a man fell forward from his seat in cardiac arrest and had barely slumped to the floor before a virtual stampede of doctors rushed to his aid. I have been on an Air France flight over the Atlantic when the classic formula was shouted by a flight attendant—in both French and English, no less— and was unable to get to the patient's side because three alert physicians were already hovering over her by the time I had dashed to her section of the airplane. Those were moments of pride in my profession, but they don't make up for the few others. The few others should never have happened.

Cardiac episodes come in a variety of forms. Some are arrests, some are heart attacks from which recovery takes place, and some prove to be not really cardiac at all. Many do not end the way my first one did. And there are some that are actually funny, even ridiculous. Of these, I have had a few experiences.

In the summer of 1994, my actress wife was playing Mistress Quickly in a production of *The Merry Wives of Windsor* at the Hudson Valley Shakespeare Festival in Garrison, New York. The play was performed in a huge four-hundred-seat tent whose single open side faced a magnificent sloping landscape just across the river from West Point. On opening night, moments before Mistress Quickly was to appear in her big first-act scene, those ominous and too-familiar words burst forth in the stentorian baritone of the stage manager: "Is there a doctor in the house?"

The cause of the disturbance was a woman in late middle age, leaning forward in her seat and clutching the front of her dress as though experiencing chest pain. Both of us being situated in the first row and separated by only about fifteen feet, I was able to get to her side immediately, only to have her whisper at me that she was so embarrassed by all the attention that she just wanted to get out of the theater. Because our seats were adjacent to the open side, her wish was easily accommodated by our slowly walking together a distance of no more than a dozen yards until we were concealed behind the tent's heavy canvas.

By the time I had helped her to lie down on the grass, another physician had come forth from the audience. He proved to be a cardiac anesthesiologist on the staff of the Columbia-Presbyterian Medical Center. Fate could not have been more kind. Other than to say some comforting words, not much could be done until the quickly summoned ambulance came (we would later learn that our patient had had a relatively mild coronary), but my experienced colleague's presence was reassuring. Being from the town, the ambulance driver knew not to use his siren near the theater, so the play was able to proceed after only a few minutes' delay. But I did miss my wife's first big scene.

There were forty performances of *The Merry Wives of Windsor* that season, of which I saw three more. On the final evening of the run, I returned for the last time. As usual, my younger children, a few guests, and I had an early picnic dinner on the spacious, beautifully manicured lawn. As we wandered over the grounds before going in to take our seats, my attention was caught by a corpulent man in his twenties who had obviously overindulged in both food and grog. His face was plethoric, his belly bulged against his belt, and he was staggering just a bit as he made his way toward the tent in the company of a displeased young woman who must have been his date. I was afraid he would vomit before he got there.

The final performance began. At precisely the same instant as the episode on opening night, that same powerful voice roared out those same words. Whatever the cause, I knew that I would once again miss the big speech. I quickly scanned the audience and found that cause: it was the overindulgent young man, standing at his seat and retching, his face a purplish gob of distress. He was a thoroughly repulsive sight. Though I knew that his problem was only indigestion, I also knew that I should go to him. I was frustrated, furious, and disgusted, all at the same time.

The theater had become dead quiet at the sound of the stage manager's booming summons. Only the twittering of evening birds could be heard, as everyone sat in stunned silence. I took a determined—if reluctant—step toward my duty, but not before a barnyard profanity escaped from my jangled thoughts and, at the same time, from my incautious lips. The words came forth not much louder than an ordinary spoken sentence, but in that hushed space of acoustic magnifications, the mute air was shattered by the exclamation of a doctor so fed up that he couldn't contain himself: *"Oh shit!"* The sound of it roared outward to fill that entire canvas-wrapped enclosure, so empty of any other human voice. I was sure the expletive could be heard for miles around. Its reverberation escaped through the open end of the tent and echoed back into the theater from the surrounding hills, or so it seemed to its mortified declaimer. Gone was any semblance of medical dignity, as the entire cast—even those standing in the wings—began to laugh uproariously, joined immediately by the audience. The stricken young man rushed from his place with both hands clapped tightly against his mouth, hiccuping until he disappeared behind the tent. A moment later, the loathsome sound of loud vomiting could be heard, emanating through the canvas from the spot to which he had fled. He never returned, and that seemed to suit his date just fine. She stayed and enjoyed the rest of the performance, which had been halted only long enough for my cussing and his puking. I didn't miss a single Shakespearian iamb.

WRITING

Nowadays it is impossible to have one's name on a book or two without being deluged with questions from well-meaning people, wanting to know how the craft of writing is done. I wish I had an answer.

Other than its association with that word itself—"craft"—writing would seem to have little in common with surgery, the job that occupied my days and nights for almost four decades. Surgery is an exercise in precision, a tour de force of organized teamwork, and a tribute to the supremacy of planning and forethought. No matter the variations, unexpected findings, or even occasional mishaps that may be encountered in its performance, the essence of the undertaking is to bring every irregularity back into the preconceived arc of intent, so that the trajectory goes directly toward its necessary goal. The surgeon attempts to replicate a perfection that can be reached only by removing himself from the emotion of the moment. Writing, or at least writing as I do it, is impossible without an exhilarating sense of freedom that carries author and reader to unexpected places. For each of them, it is a solitary journey of discovery, unique each time it is made. Its very substance is emotion.

Yet I am not alone in my attraction to the polarity between writing and surgery. For those of us who practice both, the confining strictures of surgery are made acceptable and even comforting by the uncontrolled thinking through which we are carried along while writing. Writing lifts me up and wafts me around in that sublime detachment from the here and now, and even from the directed goal that stabilizes my mind while I am operating or facing a clinical decision at the bedside. And surgery provides a groundwork of structure and substantiality that connects me to the place from which I may safely abscond while writing, knowing that its predictable refuge awaits me when I return. These are two different forms of excitement, between which I don't know if I have ever achieved a balance. But I have certainly had a lot of fun.

It is hardly false modesty to point out that I am not really a writer. I am a surgeon who has been at his calling for a very long time and carries a sensory load so deeply buried by layers of accumulated experiences that he barely knows that most of it exists. Even "barely" is excessive—at any moment all but small bits of it are hidden and seemingly inaccessible. In this, I come to the work of writing in much the same way as would a lawyer, a businessman, a teacher, or a diplomat; I come to the work in much the same way as would a butcher, a baker, a candlestick maker, or even a Bowery bum. Though life has shown each of us a different scene, we are alike in having analyzed what we've experienced again and again, always in the light of everything we have subsequently undertaken and undergone. And much of this harvesting of new meanings has taken place without our being aware of it.

Even the least introspective of us cannot escape a decades-long accumulation of impressions, gestalts, weltanschauungs, philosophies, and musings on the human condition. Although our recollection may be distorted as we view events through the lens of later times and later patterns of thinking, the passage of time adds to our ability to make sense of them, even if they have somewhat lost their shape in the vast caverns of a complex emotional life. Our impressions of the past are carried at a mostly unconscious level, as feelings, stored images of varying degrees of sharpness, unstructured ruminations, and other inchoate shapes. The past melds with the present and waits to be rediscovered and rethought.

Emotion is the closest thing to truth that the human mind possesses. When we attempt to articulate it to others, emotion leads to an unstructured thought, which leads to a structured thought, which leads to the language required to express it. Though some will disagree, I believe it is ultimately the transmission of emotion that is the root of the distinctive form of communication we call literature. If we let it, writing brings everything forward. But in order for this to happen, writing must be done in an atmosphere of unhampered spontaneity, of free association like that so valued by our psychoanalytic brethren.

When Aldous Huxley asserted that good writing is "free association, artistically controlled," he was not far from William Wordsworth's description of poetry as "emotion recollected in tranquillity." To write—whether it takes the form of poetry or prose, fiction or nonfiction—is to let the words take form from the thought brought forth by feeling. Nathaniel Hawthorne took the process a bit further: "The greatest merit of style is, of course, to make the words absolutely disappear into the thought." But the feeling must come first.

The retrieving from those deep places can be done only by the uncensored mind allowing itself to feel the uncensored emotion. While letting this process flow, one must not think of style or even of content—what will out will out, and it must be followed wherever it leads. Style, too, will follow. This is as true of fiction, and even of the writing of history or opinion, as it is of poetry. Only in technical papers is it to be avoided, or so say the mahatmas of the professional journals—but I sometimes wonder whether here and there a place shouldn't be found for it.

And so, when asked how I write, I say that there is no real method but to have faith in the unconscious, a reply that almost always leaves questing interrogators unsatisfied. And I do trust my unconscious to find the way, and even to guide my writing toward thematic cohesion. It has been my invariable habit, whether composing a chapter like this one or a full-length book, to pay no mind to the totality of its structure. I have never made an outline; I have never thought about the ending while writing the beginning; I have never planned chapter 4 while working on chapter 3; I have never considered what themes or lessons are to be drawn from the piece, preferring that they make themselves apparent to the reader (and to me) as the work unfolds.

Truth be told, I have never planned so much as a sentence ahead. To me, writing is like being borne along on a Ouija board—it takes me where it will.

It may astonish some readers to be told that every piece I have ever written has somehow, willy-nilly, found its own beginning, middle, and end. My conscious mind has had no hand in this, ever. The writing has happened by itself. It seems always to find the shape, the message, and the symmetry that make it a whole. The unconscious may seem to meander, but it knows where it is going and precisely how to get there— I refer here not to *my* unconscious alone but to everyone's—if people would only let it do what it wants. I suspect that far more writers follow its path than many readers realize. Percy Bysshe Shelley understood this better than most. He wrote, "The very mind which directs the hands in formation is incapable of accounting to itself for the origin, the gradations, or the media of the process."

And the unconscious does something else that a writer eventually gets used to, but not before it has flabbergasted him again and again with its incalculable power. It unearths information that he does not know he has. It brings back memories he would otherwise have no way of recalling. Names, facts, entire scenarios come forward as though they had been awaiting the summons to this moment, called up by the power of untrammeled free association. This process is not one that needs thinking about: it happens by itself, is brought forth by the very act of writing. One thought leads ineluctably to another and yet another, and before a page is completed a pattern has emerged that is beyond anything anticipated at the outset. Whatever intent the writer may have had when he began often has no relation to the final product. The Ouija board is a miraculous vehicle.

And what comes forth is not only information. As thought forms, it merges into opinion, and before he is through, the writer not infrequently finds that he has propounded a philosophy that he had no idea was forming in his mind. I have never written a book in which a coherent point of view that was either nebulous or quite unknown to me didn't appear on the page as though I'd been its champion for years. Reading a completed manuscript, I have been taken aback by worldviews I proposed of which I had no forethought, which I hardly remembered having recorded on the paper. They might have been written by someone else, except that they seem to give precise expression to my own convictions. I have been brought to tears by stories of my own childhood experiences told in a voice that I recognize as my own, and yet I cannot clearly recall having written them.

These are among the reasons that I always encourage people to try writing. What better way to find out about oneself, to bring back memories and the sweet pain of nostalgia, to give form to ideas previously uncertain, and to discover truths that would otherwise remain hidden? What better way to see that the events in which we have partaken are recognizable to those who read about them, even if in a different form? What better way to come to the realization that the more one reveals his most intimate experiences and thoughts, the more he is expressing universal themes, understood by every reader? There is joy in this, and an indescribable sense of having brought meaning to the events of everyday life.

It might be thought that virtually all the foregoing refers to autobiography or memoir, but that wouldn't be correct. I believe the writer belongs on every page he writes, whether he is speaking directly about his experiences and his views or is present only as the voice through which information is conveyed. Unless one is making an overt effort to imitate another's patterns of composition—an uncomfortable thing to attempt, which completely inhibits the spontaneity of the unconscious—the very sound of his sentences is unique to the author. His style is formed by everything he has ever read, everything he has ever experienced, everything he has ever thought. It is uniquely his. It brings a distinctive quality to his work and is perhaps the most important of the factors that make him different from any other writer. Wanting to be or not, he is there on the page.

Every essayist, of course, knows this. But so does every other thoughtful person who has ever put words on paper for anything but the driest of technical articles. Michel de Montaigne said it best, some four centuries ago: *"Je suis moi-même la matière de mon livre"* ("I am myself the substance of my book"). Every bit of fiction, nonfiction, and poetry has been produced by the only man or woman who could have written it. Each of its sentences should proclaim that fact.

*   *   *

But all of this pertains to any writing. The point of this book is to muse about my experience of a career in medicine, so I will look at the special characteristics of medical writing. There is the factor of technical language, of course, and the ever-present danger that readers will see themselves in any clinical situation that might be described. Not much can be done about the latter, but the former is easily handled by one or both of two strategies. The etymology of words may be provided so their medical usage becomes clear, or the authors may avoid such terms entirely, eschewing the medical for plain English. Medical terminology is, after all, only a form of shorthand, and it is not always necessary.

This aspect of medical writing is shared by any literature that deals with complex matters—from philosophy to physics—in which an arcane language of experts has grown up. But there is a major concern that is unique to doctors writing about medicine: the need for confidentiality in the information they disclose about their patients.

The first and most obvious rule is never to use any person's actual name unless given permission to do so. If other circumstances can be disguised without prejudicing the verisimilitude of the narrative, this, too, must be done. But it is necessary to be extremely wary in such things. A medical case history by its very nature is a story in which the altering of a few apparently small details may have a significant effect on the judgments to be made or the lessons to be drawn. The finest distinctions of fact, or the most intimate characteristics of a patient and the course of his disease, may carry clues to the entire point of the story. Some of this material can be sufficiently unlovely that there might be hesitancy in disclosing it. But in clinical descriptions, there is no substitute for absolute truth, and often no substitute for the depiction of grim or grimy images.

And there's the rub. The absolute truth in all of its stark clinical reality may be perceived by the patient as a violation of confidentiality, even when names and places are changed. What is to be done about this, short of so modifying the story that it loses its meaning?

Another way to put this question is the form in which it was asked of me not long ago by a young physician-writer, a man deeply concerned with the ethical consequences of such narratives. Even when the patient has been rendered completely unrecognizable, is there a violation of trust if no permission is sought, or if the man or woman has died? Is there a violation of trust when permission has actually been granted but the patient has no idea of the detailed scrutiny to which he and his disease will be subjected by the physician? Does the physician's need to tell a story that may have wide—even life-changing—implications for his readers justify such a breach of confidentiality? Is it, in fact, a breach of confidentiality at all? Further, since clinical descriptions routinely appear in standard medical journals, usually without permission, is there really a difference between such writings and those of a more literary nature? As my correspondent so trenchantly summarized the conundrum: "To whom does the story belong?"

Many will disagree with my response, but I submit it for reflection by all who would undertake such writings. What I propose here would seem to follow naturally from the methods by which I have suggested that truth may be found in all forms of literary work.

The act of writing is a process that enables us to recall things as they were experienced while they were happening—especially if they are long-ago events—in the light of later years. It permits us to articulate both how those events appear to our minds at the moment of recording and what lessons they may teach. Writing makes it possible to find out what we think, often for the first time. It is a process that will be totally honest if we are willing to feel those emotions that are coming forth from preserved memory and to put them down on paper uncensored. While this process is taking place, there can be no consideration of ethics, confidentiality, or even loyalty to participants. There is only the reality of what the writer feels to be the truth of what he is describing. In short, what I do is change the names and never consider the consequences that may result from my efforts to achieve the essential truth.

Others have written that all writers ultimately betray those who are their subjects. But they would betray themselves were it otherwise—and their readers too. Writing is not an exercise in discretion; it is an exercise in seeking the clues to our lives. In this sense, the story belongs to the storyteller, because the storyteller is the truth seeker. At the risk of appearing lofty, I believe that the storyteller is also the person communicating the truth to the world, perhaps to posterity. A distinguished medical historian, now long dead, once told me that doctors are the only real philosophers, because only doctors know how people actually behave. Perhaps that is an overstatement, but the practice of medicine has been my key to understanding the way we live, and I use it to search for the reality of the human condition.

ROBBING GRAVES

The body in question belonged to a nine-year-old girl named Ruth Sprague. It had been stolen from its grave by a certain Roderick Clow on the night after she was buried in 1846 and then taken to the office of a local physician, Dr. P. M. Armstrong, where it was secretly dissected—anatomized—in the name of medical science. Along with the quatrain, the despised names of Clow and Armstrong were engraved on the tombstone for posterity to read, that their shameful deed not be forgotten. Also engraved there is the remarkable statement that "her mutilated remains were obtained and deposited here."

Recovery of whatever was left of a clandestinely disinterred and anatomized corpse was a rarity, and there is no way of knowing just how the residuum of Ruth came to be buried in that place. Nor does there appear to be any evidence that either Clow or Armstrong was punished in any way for the theft or the dissection. They very likely went free, because only in the previous decade had anatomy laws been written to criminalize such desecrations, and even then their main objective was not to punish but to provide a steady supply of teaching material to medical schools. These statutes made available the bodies of the executed and the unknown, as well as those of people for whom no burial provisions had been made (certain paupers, for example), but

the punitive measures against illegal disinterment went generally un-
enforced.

When Clow set out on his grisly mission that night, he was,
whether knowingly or not, engaging in a line of work in which others
had achieved a degree of dubious fame and even a kind of immortality.
Not a few of his predecessors' exploits appear like unsightly blots on
the pages of medical history, staining the images of some of the greatest anatomists and surgeons of all time. Many prominent teachers of
surgery not only sponsored these unsavory doings but led expeditions
of corporeal salvage themselves. Robert Liston of University College,
London, who did the first European operation using ether in the very
year of Ruth Sprague's postmortem dismemberment, was known to
plunder cemeteries in the company of a notorious grave robber named
Crouch. In one twice-told tale of Liston's adventures, he and Crouch
argued over the rights to a grave site with a young surgeon in training, Mowbray Thomson, who finally carried the field by pulling out
a pistol and threatening to kill the powerfully built surgeon. Liston
and his henchman wisely retreated, thus avoiding the possibility of
joining the disputed corpse as supine subjects of Thomson's scientific
curiosity.

Human dissection was rare before the middle of the sixteenth century
because medical theory was based on the concept of the imbalance of
the four internal fluids, or humors; a detailed knowledge of anatomy
was deemed unnecessary. The few textbook illustrations of organs
were symbolic rather than accurate. Once or twice a year, medical
schools provided a hurried public dissection of a cadaver—usually
done by teachers who knew little more than their students—but only
to provide a general idea of what the inside of a patient looked like.
Things gradually began to change after 1543, the year of Andreas
Vesalius's publication of his magnum opus, *De humani corporis fabrica*,
the first complete textbook based on the dissection of human bodies.
Vesalius's ability to obtain cadavers was enhanced by a bull that
had been issued by Pope Sixtus IV in 1482, revoking the church's
centuries-old prohibitions against human dissection and allowing local

bishops to provide assent—and usually to provide the bodies too. The corpses of criminals, of the unknown or unclaimed dead, and of those who died intestate were by this means made available to physicians and artists. Without the papal bull, Leonardo da Vinci and Michelangelo would never have learned so much about the form and function of the major muscles. No such provision existed in Protestant countries.

By the end of the eighteenth century, medical theory had advanced sufficiently that proper instruction of aspiring doctors was impossible without a reliable and plentiful source of cadavers. In England and Scotland, this presented a problem for the new breed of hospital-based clinicians and pathologists, whose research demanded more corpses than the few made available by executions. Not only that, independent schools for anatomy instruction were beginning to crop up in Edinburgh and London. Because they competed for students and won them by providing their dissecting tables with an uninterrupted flow of dead citizens, their need for bodies seemed endless. Medical professors in America, although they lagged far behind their European colleagues in both science and instruction, were having similar difficulties obtaining cadavers.

Wherever there is an expanding need for some new product, entrepreneurs of one kind or another are likely to appear, eager to fill it. The ever-growing demand for newly dead and still intact human flesh was no exception. By the end of the eighteenth century, an entirely new profession had sprung up in the sceptered isle, and practitioners were also beginning to appear in the New World. They were variously called grave robbers, resurrectionists (for their skills at raising the dead), and sack-'em-up men (for their habit of depositing the unearthed bodies in large cloth bags for delivery to customers).

Their methods soon took on a degree of standardization. As is true in all businesses, when ambitious young people working for a firm leave it to go out on their own, they continue to use the techniques their mentors have taught them. As it was necessary to work quickly and leave as little evidence of disturbance as possible, a particularly expeditious sequence of steps evolved. A hole would be dug over only the part of the coffin lid that covered the prospective specimen's head and shoulders; all of the removed sod would be deposited on a canvas to prevent it from marring the adjacent grass. The digging was done with specially prepared daggers of sharpened wood to avoid the clang that rings out when metal strikes stones. When the lid was reached, two broad hooks of iron were attached to its upper portion; sacking was packed over it to deaden the sound of breaking wood; and a quick, forcible jerk upward cracked it open. Having removed the short segment of broken lid, the body thieves would drag the corpse out head first, remove its burial clothes, and return them to the coffin. After carefully replacing the sod, they would then sack up the body and at some point in the night deliver it to the open-pursed assistant of one or another generous prince of medicine.

As might be supposed, the sort of men attracted to this kind of work were not admirable. In the words of Henry Lonsdale, a contemporary Scottish teacher of anatomy, "Nothing was too base for them to do. Their countenances betrayed a sinister expression, and their dress, always shabby, neither resembled the artisan nor the lowest tradesman; they were non-descripts in person, as they were in character." But thanks to the medical men, they were nondescripts with plenty of money in their pockets. In 1828, the police estimated that two hundred of them were plying their lucrative trade in London; ten made it their sole occupation.

As the practices became better known and more reliable, the surgeon customers increasingly separated themselves from the dirty work, using students or assistants as intermediaries with the nefarious tradesmen. This less direct form of complicity not only eased their pangs of conscience but also made them less vulnerable to retribution. The few prominent surgeons of the time had vast incomes and were willing to pay handsomely (Sir Astley Cooper, London's leading surgeon from about 1810 to perhaps 1830, is reliably said to have earned £100,000 in 1816, when a pound was worth five dollars and a seven-course meal could be had for less than ten shillings). In all, it was a tidy arrangement, fulfilling the needs of both purchaser and procurer.

But it was difficult and dangerous work. Cemeteries were patrolled by armed watchmen; families kept guard at the graves of the newly buried or hired toughs to do it for them. Many resurrectionists were badly beaten, and a few were killed. Some of the more enterprising members of the profession invented schemes that kept them out of harm's way or that helped them circumvent the cagelike steel housing, called a mortsafe, that some wealthy families took to putting over a grave immediately after the funeral.

The most common way to avoid working the graveyard shift, as it were, was to be constantly on the alert for people, especially among the poor, who were dying without friends to claim their bodies. No sooner had the final breath been taken than the sack-'em-up man would appear at the house or hospital with a lachrymose look on his face and declare between racking sobs that he was a bereaved relative. Having claimed the body, he would take it on a horse-drawn cart or some similar conveyance to the usual destination, to be used for the usual purpose.

Such stratagems required more thespian skill, though, than all but a very few of these men possessed. As families became more watchful and the competition for good specimens accordingly increased, a few of the more daring resurrectionists devised schemes that might be said to have anticipated by a century the basis upon which Henry Ford's River Rouge plant was conceived: to control the entire process of manufacture from raw materials to delivery. What this meant was the conversion of a perfectly healthy man or woman into a flawless cadaver made ready for immediate use—in a word, murder.

The lure of earning as much as thirty pounds per bag without risking life or limb had proved too tempting for several of the more barbarous resurrectionists. Surgeons and teachers of anatomy, desperate for specimens (and none too scrupulous themselves), turned a blind eye when they began to notice that an occasional corpse bore no evidence of any pathological condition that might have caused death. But more principled observers were horrified by the turn of events. *The Lancet*, which had long been crusading for proper laws to regulate anatomy instruction and the procurement of bodies, made the situation public in an editorial of January 3, 1820: "We have ourselves, within a recent period, seen bodies brought into the dissecting room in this metropolis, exhibiting none of the appearances usually found on the bodies of persons who had died from disease, but with all the indications presented by the bodies of men who had died within a few hours, and in a state of perfect health."

In spite of such revelations, the anatomy murders continued and even became more frequent. The most notorious of the perpetrators were two Irishmen named William Burke and William Hare, who contrived to kill at least sixteen of the citizens of Edinburgh in a twelve-month period ending on Halloween night of 1828, all in the name of medical science and free enterprise. Although not previously noted for particularly fine intellectual gifts, these two louts designed an ingenious method of corpse production. Their modus operandi was to ply a subject—usually a lonely, frail, elderly woman—with gin until she passed out, whereupon the ferretlike Hare would stop her mouth and nose with his bony fingers while the hydrant-shaped Burke sat on her chest. This form of suffocation left no suspicious marks, was virtually foolproof, and entailed no physical risk to the two creative industrialists. The practice has, in fact, been memorialized in the form of a transitive verb in the name of its more active participant, defined in the *Oxford English Dictionary* as follows: *burke: kill (a person) to sell the body for dissection; suffocate or strangle secretly.* It is said that the hallmark of lasting fame is to be remembered as the eponym for an uncapitalized word (*watt* or *boycott*, for example). If so, the name of William Burke is destined to endure.

Burke and Hare found an eager customer in the person of Dr. Robert Knox, the proprietor of a private anatomy school patronized by medical students at the University of Edinburgh. With such a steady patron, the two adventurers were rollicking in the success of their commercial venture, when it was suddenly halted by the discovery of the body of an old woman, Margaret Docherty, hidden under a pile of straw in the seedy rooming house where they lived with their two slatternly mistresses. Hare turned King's evidence against Burke, who was hanged in a riotous ceremony witnessed by more than twenty thousand jubilant onlookers as though it were carnival day (which, in the literal sense, it was, considering the origin of that word from the Latin *carne vale*, "flesh farewell," of Shrove Tuesday or Mardi Gras). By order of the court, Burke's corpse was then turned over to Alexander

Monro, a professor of anatomy at the University of Edinburgh, to be publicly dissected. Over the next two days, some forty thousand people filed past Dr. Monro's laboratory table to assure themselves that the executed fiend was getting his just desserts. What many must have known was that Monro himself was a regular sack-'em-up patron.

The exposure of Burke and Hare's villainy called public attention to the existence of anatomy murder far more effectively than had the restrained editorial in *The Lancet*. Yet no laws were enacted until the citizenry was aroused by another violent crime. On November 5, 1831, three thuggish men tried to sell the body of a fourteen-year-old Italian immigrant boy to the dissecting room porter of King's College Hospital in London. The porter, more principled than most, thought the corpse bore signs of violence. He reported this to one of the anatomy instructors, who did an autopsy and confirmed that the boy's neck had been broken. The trial at the Old Bailey resulted in the conviction of all three murderers, two of whom were subsequently hanged and dissected, while the third was sentenced to transportation to Australia.

All hell now broke loose. There were public demands for reform; even some of the resurrectionists' best customers suddenly discovered a devout righteousness they had never before recognized in themselves. No less a surgical personage than Sir Astley himself appeared before a parliamentary hearing and declared in the ringing tones (his voice has been described in the reminiscences of admiring students as "silvery") that he usually reserved for the lecture hall at Guy's Hospital Medical School, "There is no person, let his situation in life be what it may, whom, if I were disposed to dissect, I could not obtain!" This bold admission—and statements like it uttered by others in Cooper's situation—struck terror into the hearts of its listeners, and they responded in August 1832 by passing the law that became known as the Anatomy Act. This piece of legislation provided for the appointment of medical inspectors to supervise every phase of anatomy teaching and the procurement of bodies, which were not to be delivered to a school unless one of these officials was present. While it did not provide for a steady source of cadavers, the law radically changed the atmosphere in which they were obtained. Also, it paved the way for later enactments allowing for the actual willing of bodies for dissection and their voluntary assignment by family members, thereby removing much of the public perception that there was something degrading about being anatomized.

But as long as provision for instructional cadavers remained imperfect, grave robbing would continue, albeit less frequently. Many are the tales of sordid adventure in which the spiritual descendants of the resurrectionists figure as the main characters, in both Great Britain and the United States. The unearthing of Ruth Sprague was a case in point. Decades would pass before a steady supply of honestly obtained specimens became generally available. In this twenty-first century, when anatomy is often taught with the aid of computerized representations and surgeons can learn their craft in virtual reality, it is hard to believe that barely a century and a half ago, doctors and medical students consorted so freely with criminals in the pursuit of learning.

MIND, BODY, AND THE DOCTOR

It was known by every charlatan who sold bottles of foul-tasting green elixir from the back of a horse-drawn wagon; it was known by Anton Mesmer and all the other poseurs who invented one or another of the historical array of mystical therapies based on the gullibility of the afflicted and the merely nervous; it was known by high priests, shamans, and witch doctors; it was even known by Hippocrates, Galen, and the other founders of the supposedly nonsubjective Western medical tradition. I suspect that such as faith healers, homeopaths, and chiropractors, in their deepest self-reflective moments, admit it into their conscious thoughts. Why don't today's ultrasophisticated avatars of scientific medicine pay it the tribute it deserves? The authority of the physician is a powerful weapon against disease.

For millennia, that truth has been put into words in various ways. Its most direct statement may be found in the second-century-C.E. works of Galen, the Greek physician whose writings dominated medical thought from the Roman period until perhaps the seventeenth century: "He cures most successfully in whom the people have the most confidence." Galen's comment is frequently quoted (though always as if proclaiming a philosophical notion to be pondered, not as a possible therapeutic strategy). The Hippocratic literature had said much the same thing half a millennium earlier, emphasizing between the lines a patient's wish to please a doctor whom he admires: "Some patients, though conscious that their condition is perilous, recover their health simply through their contentment with the goodness of the physician."

The concept of pleasing is inherent in the so-called placebo effect, nowadays much discussed by physicians of a humanistic bent but deemed a confusing nuisance in the data-driven evaluation of drug efficacy insisted upon by today's all-too-rational biomedical establishment. The word "placebo"—Latin for "I will please"—refers to a physician's inclination to prescribe for a needful patient even though he knows that the medication has no active ingredients. He thereby pleases the patient by fulfilling his expectation that something will be done. In turn, the patient pleases the doctor by recovering, thereby fulfilling *his* expectation that some good will come of the transaction.

There are skilled physicians who pooh-pooh such therapeutic ventures as so much hocus-pocus, unworthy of their profession. Yet other physicians study the results of what would appear to their colleagues as clinical legerdemain and report the most astonishing outcomes in people so treated. The frequency of beneficial effects of placebos ranges from approximately one in five to almost three in five, depending on the way the study is carried out and the criteria by which success is measured.

Yet those of us who have seen the power of the placebo effect must now contend with its statistical "debunking" a few years ago, by two researchers attached to the Department of Medical Philosophy and Clinical Theory at the University of Copenhagen (at least until other debunkers debunk the Danes). After millennia of what they dismiss as mere "anecdotal evidence," such a report can hardly negate an experienced physician's awe at a phenomenon that might impress even a dispassionate biometrician, would he or she ever to venture within range of a real patient. Clinicians who would discard common sense and simple observation on the basis of one study should be reminded of Philosophy and Theory's long history of leading medicine astray. As the man said when his wife caught him in bed with another woman, "This is not what it looks like! Are you going to believe *me* or your eyes?" Not until the seventeenth century, when doctors began to rely less on the theories of philosophers and the advocates of all-embracing theories, and more on the evidence of their own eyes at the bedside and in the laboratory, was real progress made in understanding the basis upon which the sick might be healed.

In 1937, at the annual meeting of the American College of Physicians, Dr. W. R. Houston gave a lecture entitled "The Doctor Himself as Therapeutic Agent." The subject was the placebo effect. Dr. Houston's use of the term was not restricted to inactive prescriptions but included the entire range of that complex set of interactions that has long been known as the doctor-patient relationship:

> The great lesson, then, of medical history is that the placebo has always been the norm of medical practice. In the large view, we are forced to realize that [physicians'] learning was a learning in how to deal with men. Their skill was a skill in dealing with the emotions of men. They themselves were the therapeutic agents by which cures were effected. Their therapeutic procedures, whether they were inert or whether they were dangerous, were placebos, symbols by which their patients' faith and their own was sustained.

Scholars of the history of therapeutics would very likely go Dr. Houston one further, by correcting his use of the past tense. In 1937, there was still far too little that the average doctor could scientifically do for the average patient with the average complaint. Until antibiotics became generally available after World War II, the likelihood of an individual's being helped by the pharmacologic effects of a doctor's treatment was less than fifty-fifty. Even so, the vast majority of people seeking medical aid recovered from their illnesses.

The most obvious reason for such a salubrious state of affairs is the same one for which the medical profession (and the practitioner of every form of nonscientific healing as well, from ayurveda to amulets) has always taken credit, namely that the great majority of illnesses get better by themselves, including those with real pathology demonstrable by microscopic or chemical means. Such is the inherent stability of the molecular coping mechanisms of all living organisms that a return to a baseline of normal functioning is the response to be expected almost every time unless the body's defenses are overwhelmed. Such overwhelming is what occurs when a malignancy or massive infection has become well established or when the stabilizing tendencies have lost a sufficient quantity of their inherent ability to cope, as takes place with the incursions of advanced aging.

The healing of any disease involves a complex of factors, but all depend on those inborn corrective forces that fend off the threats against continuing viability to which each of our 75 trillion cells is exposed every instant of our lives. The purpose of medical therapy is to abet those defenses. It may accomplish its ends by removing the threat itself (cancer surgery or antibiotics are examples); strengthening the body's own protective mechanisms or replacing them when they are deficient or absent (transfusion for blood loss or insulin for diabetes); simply tiding the body over until its own recovery is sufficient to deal with the ravages of the disease (respiratory intubation or intravenous fluids); or a combination of several of these means.

But the way in which the body combines its own mobilization of forces with a physician's therapies remains obscure. Identical treatments seem to affect individual patients differently, even when their burden of disease appears similar. Researchers in the new field of pharmacogenomics claim that they will soon uncover the DNA-entangled reasons for such differences and treat them with agents designer-made to personalize the biochemical assault on sickness. Such genetically guided therapy will be a great step forward, but I am certain that it is not the entire answer to individual variations in response. It does not, for example, address the variations elicited by different physicians or medical centers when treating the same disease in large and seemingly homogeneous groups of patients, where the size of the population sample would compensate for individual genetic or other organic variations. Moreover, anyone who has long been a regular participant in the weekly or monthly conferences held by a community of physicians—within a hospital staff, for example—has observed that certain members claim and can support by statistics the efficacy of therapies that have less happy outcomes in the hands of their colleagues of similar abilities in the same institution. For other diseases and other therapies, other members of the staff may be the ones with better results.

Then there are the observations of what might be called a more mystical sort. These include the occasional patient who survives a terminal disease for a period beyond all expert predictions, long enough, for example, to see a son or daughter graduate from college; or another who refuses to die until a beloved face can be looked upon once more, even when a delay of days or longer is necessary beyond the prognostications of every skilled observer. For several years, as an informal test of a general thesis resulting from decades of subjective impressions concerning the effect of holidays on death rates, I have monitored the obituary lists of my local newspaper, the *New Haven Register*, distributed throughout an area in which more than six hundred thousand people live. Almost always, the number of deaths has shrunk dramatically before Christmas, rising precipitously when the holiday is past. Similar findings have been described by others, for similar situations. In Israel, for example, such holiday-related accounts are said to be commonplace and have been reported in medical journals.

Though none of this is attributable to the interventions of doctors, it does speak to a phenomenon more universal and therefore even more worthy of investigation: the effect of thoughts, both conscious and unconscious, on the body's response to disease. Galen, the Hippocratic authors, and the other early physicians who wrote about such things very likely believed that the psyche, an immeasurable force beyond human ability to comprehend, acted in some way on the strictly corporeal aspects of a patient to bring such effects about. "Psyche," derived from the Greek word for "soul" or "spirit," is derived from an Indo-European root that pertains to breathing—thus reflecting the ancient belief that the supernal atmosphere of the cosmos, or macrocosm, is inhaled with his first breath by the microcosm that is a man ("psyche," in fact, has commonly been used synonymously with "pneuma," referring to a notion of something similar to air). It was the mystical power of the psyche, therefore, that was believed to effect or at least affect the bodily changes caused by the mind. Even the Hippocratics, whose major contribution to medical theory was the separation of natural phenomena from supernatural explanations, believed in it.

In the seventeenth century, Cartesian dualism embedded ("encrusted" might be a better word) into the minds of those who would be serious thinkers the dogma that mind and body are distinct. Though the effects of the one on the other have always been observed, it was thought that such occurrences were beyond the ability of conjecture or research to explain, since mind is a nonphysical concept and body is a palpable structure. But there is, in fact, no duality. Mind is a function of the organic processes of the brain and almost certainly of the rest of the body as well. In this it is like digestion or assimilation of nutrients, which until the early nineteenth century appeared to be just as inscrutable as thought or mind seem today. Our physical and chemical structure determines digestion; digestion in turn influences our physical and chemical structure. In the same way, body determines mind and mind influences body. It is only a matter of time before the unity of mind and body—so apparent from observation—is demonstrated in scientific terms and their interdependence elucidated. And when that has been accomplished, we will have biophysical explanations for such phenomena as the frequency of the interrelationship sometimes observed between a patient's expectations or hopes, for example, and the outcome of his disease—and even the occasional person's apparent ability to change the course of an illness when all scientific treatment seems to have failed.

In the early 1960s a group of internists and scientists at the University of Rochester demonstrated a connection between the onset of lymphatic cancer, or lymphoma, and a patient's having had a major personal loss within the previous six months, such as the death of a loved one, divorce, or the loss of a home or job. Stimulated by these findings (which until then had been recognized by many physicians but never studied in any systematic way), they and others began applying the rigorous methods of laboratory and statistical research to investigate such phenomena. The result was the founding of an entirely new area of study, which was given the name "psychoneuroimmunology." Though a jawbreaker of a word, "psychoneuroimmunology" can be broken down into its constituent parts, to reveal that the discipline's purpose is to study the relationship among psyche, brain, nervous system, endocrine gland secretions, immune mechanisms, and response to disease. It involves the bench research of neuroscientists, molecular biologists, immunologists, and physiologists as well as the more clinical and patient-based work of internists, endocrinologists, social scientists, and psychologists. Their goal is to learn how the mind and the nervous system participate with the rest of the body in responding to factors in the internal and external environments, including those that affect its integrity and health.

Among those factors is the doctor himself as a therapeutic agent.

Today's healer is descended from a hoary tradition in which magic was the main—and often the only—ingredient of cure, and, knowingly or not, he or she has abandoned very little of its clinical usefulness. The specialized knowledge, the esoteric language, the symbolic stethoscope, the white coat or the scrub suit, the aura and the emotional distance from everyday life of the modern medical center—how different are these, after all, from the atmosphere of the Aesculapian temple of healing? There the white-robed priests strolled from patient to patient, murmuring incantations, laying on hands, interpreting dreams and the statements made to them by the sick, and recommending a regimen or course of therapy based on principles known only to the *Iatros*, the physician possessed of a corpus of recondite wisdom shared only with his fellows and passed down to the elect. In preserving the ancient Aesculapian symbol of healing, the snake (how very like the stethoscope's dangling tube!) entwined around the priestly staff, the priests of high-tech biomedicine confirm what is obvious from their every act in the name of the art of healing: that their authority remains to this day the most basic ingredient of their ability to cure. That authority is the foundation upon which the confidence is built, of which Galen wrote almost two thousand years ago—and it is manifest, among other ways, in a patient's wish to please the modern-day Iatros by recovering.

Every doctor has anecdotes about this kind of thing, and I have a bagful. The one to be here related is a tale I have told many times over the more than forty years since it occurred, because it was my first such experience after becoming a brand-new attending surgeon on completion of my residency training. To this day, it is the most dramatic example of Dr. Houston's thesis that I have encountered. And it also says something about the Hippocratic confidence in the therapeutic power of a physician's goodness.

The clinical case history is that of a man in his early forties who was admitted to the Yale–New Haven Hospital with empyema, a large collection of infected fluid in the left side of his chest, resulting from pneumonia. The organism causing this serious state of affairs was the staphylococcus, a bacterium largely resistant to the antibiotics available at the time. Numerous attempts to remove the thick, turbid fluid—which was in fact pus—with syringes and tubes had been unsuccessful because scarring between the lung and chest wall had loculated the noxious stuff into small compartments that could not be effectively drained. Not only that, but these multiple pockets of pus were compressing the lung, seeding the circulation with bacteria and causing extreme toxicity, with fevers reaching at least 102 degrees Fahrenheit each day. Gradually, a man who had been robustly healthy only a few weeks earlier had become a wan shadow of himself, debilitated and rapidly worsening. The outlook was grave; the senior physicians were pessimistic. As a last resort, they called for a surgeon, in the hope that fresh eyes might see a solution that had eluded them. Asked to consult, I suggested the precarious strategy of an attempt at operation to remove the cause of contamination. They quickly agreed that the only way to clean out the infected areas and free the lung was by means of the proposed hazardous surgery. I discussed the dangers of the procedure with the patient and his wife, carefully explaining our lack of remaining options. Following our discussion, I scheduled the case for two days hence, in order to leave time for certain restorative measures to be taken before I would dare undertake an operation of such magnitude. On the afternoon prior to the scheduled day, I went to see my patient on rounds and found that he was without fever for the first time since his hospital admission almost two weeks earlier. When his temperature remained normal that evening, I canceled the operation. Within a few more days it was obvious by physical findings and repeated X-ray studies that he had begun to improve. A week later, he was well enough to be discharged from the hospital. So unexplainable had been his recovery that even the most cynical clinicians had begun to use words like "miracle."

A few years later, I ran into my former patient at a wedding, and he told me why he had recovered. "I did it for Bizzozero," he said. Joe Bizzozero had been the intern assigned to this difficult case, and he had faltered not a moment in his dedication and in his certainty that our mutual patient would somehow recover, even as the odds mounted against such an outcome. In the depths of his concern and his compassion, he had spent many extra hours—including more than a few evenings when he should have been off—at the bedside of this desperately sick man edging ever closer to death, never giving up hope that a solution might be found. And he did find it—the solution was himself.

To the patient, the outcome was no miracle. Though he was a man of deep religious faith—his name was William Sloane Coffin, and he was the chaplain of Yale University—he insisted that nothing miraculous had happened. Even when pressed for his thoughts on divine intervention, he denied having any. His explanation was direct, and there was nothing of the supernatural in it. "I did it for Bizzozero," he said as if it were the most ordinary thing in the world. "I couldn't let him down."

THE GREAT BOOKS

Another damned, thick, square book! Always scribble, scribble, scribble! Eh, Mr. Gibbon?" So the Duke of Gloucester is said to have exclaimed in 1781, when Edward Gibbon presented him with a copy of the second volume of *The History of the Decline and Fall of the Roman Empire.* We have no record of the portly little scholar's response, but we may guess that he paid scant heed to the nobleman's foolishness. The first volume of his chronicle had been so astonishingly successful that Gibbon must already have suspected that his "scribbles" might be destined for literary immortality.

Since the *Iliad* and the Bible, the course of our civilization has been marked by the appearance of great books, some of which have become recently designated as Great Books. For every one of these that competes for inclusion in the so-called Western Canon, there are dozens, of equal importance to the development of our culture, that are little read or are remembered only by specialists of one sort or another. Among them are some of the landmark works in the history of medical knowledge. More than the members of any other profession or calling—except perhaps the clergy—doctors have always recorded their experiences and interpretations. They have done this primarily for instructional and archival reasons, but a by-product has been the influence of such works on the ways in which their readers think about humankind's relationship with nature. I've chosen four books, each representing a century, to illustrate the uses to which some of the greatest of medical scribblings have been put by their readers.

Today the vast majority of additions to medical knowledge are transmitted via professional journals and meetings, or even online.

The reliance on periodicals began in the middle of the nineteenth century and grew rapidly thereafter. Thus, of any advance of the twentieth century, the contribution destined to have the most profound effect on diagnosis and therapy—the discovery of the structure of DNA—was communicated in a few pages of the British scientific weekly *Nature*. That journal—along with *Science, The New England Journal of Medicine, The Lancet,* and a few others—is one of the sources to which physicians customarily turn when they seek information about the latest findings, and even the clinical implications, of biomedical research. Books, on the other hand, are more apt to be compilations of material long since reported in journals or explications of the theoretical or philosophical speculation that has always accompanied the healer's art. Since rapidity of dissemination and virtually immediate sharing have become crucial to the scientific enterprise, books are unlikely to reclaim their former importance. In some ways that is a pity. Much has been gained, but something has been lost. Gone are the literary and aesthetic qualities of the books that have marked the long road on which medicine traveled once it saw that its most fitting partner for the journey was science, not religion or superstition.

Medicine's intertwining with science began when physicians finally realized that universalizing, all-explaining theories about human biology served only to foster the misinterpretation of observed phenomena. Until then, a conflict between what was actually experienced and what the grand conceptual scheme told a physician he *should* be experiencing was always resolved in favor of the latter.

Among the most egregious examples of old-school thinking was the invention—for "invention" is precisely what it was—of a structure called the *rete mirabile* by the second-century medical mahatma, Galen. In keeping with the inherited dogma of his predecessors, Galen taught that the vital pneuma, an inscrutable airy quality that was believed to bring the life and spirit of the universe into the body, is inhaled from the surrounding cosmos. In order for intellectual activity and movement to be regulated, Galen assured his centuries of unquestioning followers, the vital pneuma had to be converted into a formulation he called *psychic* pneuma before reaching the brain. Galen claimed to have found the structure in which this process took place: a coiled network of blood vessels at the base of the skulls of the dogs, monkeys, and pigs he dissected. Never having opened the body of a human being, Galen assumed that these vessels were to be found in all mammals.

To Galen's mind—guided by the all-encompassing notions of pneuma, spirit, and the humors, and by the entire edifice of inherited cosmic philosophy that had been erected to explain the workings of nature—the discovery of such structures as the *rete mirabile* was virtually a necessity. It filled a gap in his comprehension of the grand plan set into motion by a masterful demiurge or prime mover. In fact, there was not a shred of evidence for the existence of the *rete mirabile*, in animals or elsewhere. Since Galen was virtually alone in such anatomical explorations, the few criticisms of his findings were drowned in the chorus of approval that would establish his domination of medical thought for a millennium and a half.

Thanks to a great book, Galen's seemingly indestructible temple of theory eventually crumbled into the dust of history. In August 1543, a twenty-eight-year-old professor (yes, a twenty-eight-year-old professor!) of anatomy published a remarkable volume called *De humani corporis fabrica* (*On the Workings of the Human Body*), and the world of medicine changed forever. The volume's 663 folio pages, 11 large plates, and almost 300 other illustrations were the product of the first systematic dissections of man ever published for the instruction of physicians. Eschewing the fanciful theories to which the physicians of his time were heir, Professor Andreas Vesalius of the University of Padua had meticulously dissected a series of cadavers and, influenced only by what he actually saw, had faithfully recorded his observations. He refused to be misled by errors of the past or by the grand scheme of the theoretical demiurge. In a triumphant proclamation of the new way of discovering biological reality, he urged his readers to rely only on "the book of the human body that cannot lie," exhorting them to "begin to put faith in their own not ineffectual sight and powers of reason rather than in the writings of Galen." Galen, he said, had been "deceived by his monkeys" and by his determination to marshal evidence to support the worldview he espoused. Not only was there no *rete mirabile* at the base of the brain, but some two hundred other anatomical formulations that Galen had put forward to conform with the all-embracing conceptual framework of ancient authority were also found to be erroneous.

Vesalius's was far more than a mere textbook of anatomy. Realizing that the book's publication would be one of the great turning points in the history of ideas, the young anatomist was resolved that every detail of production be as painstaking and technically peerless as his dissections. The illustrations were drawn by Jan Stephan van Calcar, a student of Titian; to find the most skilled woodblock cutters of the time, the author traveled to Venice. When all was completed, he packed the blocks and text on the backs of mules and followed them on the long, perilous journey over the Alps to Basel, where Joannes Oporinus maintained one of the finest printing establishments in Europe. The Vesalian masterpiece was a great achievement not only in the history of anatomy but also in the craft of bookmaking and in the art of pedagogy.

But the most important result of the *Fabrica*'s appearance was its underlying doctrine of reliance only on one's own experiences, unbiased by the influence of the past or by theoretical constructions based on philosophical concepts. It is by the small steps of interpreting individual observations that theories should be constructed, said Vesalius, not the other way around; observations must not be deformed by forcing them to fit into grand schemes hatched by abstract thinkers in bygone days.

That was the stance adopted in the following century by William Harvey. In 1628 he produced *Exercitatio anatomica de motu cordis et sanguinis in animalibus* (*On the Motion of the Heart and Blood in Animals*), the great book that some have called the most important contribution ever made to the study of human biology. In accordance with received wisdom, Galen had taught—and physicians still believed—that blood reached the structures of the body by a process of ebb and flow through the veins, originating in the liver. Because, according to the ancient authority's formulation, the tissues used most of the blood that reached them, the flow had to be constantly replenished by the liver. Following the example of Vesalius, Harvey decided to see for himself. His conclusion, after a series of experiments and measurements (the first time, incidentally, that quantitative evidence had been used in the study of physiology), was "that the blood is driven into a round by a circular motion . . . and lastly, that the motion and pulsation of the heart is the only cause." Flying in the face of accepted dogma, Harvey had discovered the circulation of the blood and its origin in the pumping action of the heart.

Unlike his predecessor's *Fabrica*, Harvey's *De motu cordis* is an unprepossessing little book. Its seventy-two quarto-sized pages measure five and a half by seven and a half inches and are printed in pedestrian fashion. On a shelf of medical classics, the book is hardly noticeable. But its modest appearance and its brevity are of no account: it is a kind of Gettysburg Address of medical discovery. After Harvey's finding, the value of inductive reasoning—championed in another great book of the time, Francis Bacon's *Novum organum*—became the standard of medical research and theory. Bacon's work was at the core of what has been called the Scientific Revolution of the extraordinarily productive seventeenth century. It fell to Harvey to encapsulate the entire process in his usual succinct manner by saying of Mother Nature, "[A]s long as we confer with our own eyes, and make our ascent from lesser things to higher, we shall at length be received into her closet-secrets." This was the philosophy of Vesalius, and it would be the philosophy of every important medical scientist who came after.

From the standpoint of clinical progress, the great book of the following century was one published by a man then nearing the end of a long life. In 1761, when he was seventy-nine, Giovanni Morgagni brought forth his monumental three-volume work, *De sedibus et causis morborum per anatomen indagatis* (*Seats and Causes of Diseases Investigated by Anatomy*) and in a single stroke drove the last nail into the coffin of Galen's dying theories. Consistent with earlier Greek conceptions, Galen had taught that disease resulted from an imbalance of four theoretical humors. In reporting a series of seven hundred dissections, Morgagni demonstrated that people sicken not on account of fluxes of one or another humor but because of anatomical changes within organs of the body. It was not the surfeit or deficiency of phlegm or blood or black or yellow bile that produced the symptoms associated with individual diseases but abnormalities in the tissues themselves. In referring to symptoms as "the cries of the suffering organs," Morgagni called attention to the ways in which inner pathologies might be detected by taking a history or examining a patient. Not surprisingly, *De sedibus* led to the development of routine techniques of physical examination and eventually to the invention of the stethoscope in 1816. Another medical scribbler had raised the curtain on modern techniques of diagnosis and therapeutics.

The nineteenth century was the last in which progress in healing and the general dissemination of medical knowledge were delineated primarily by great books. Though journals were being established and professional meetings were being held with increasing frequency, a number of important volumes appeared, maintaining the old landmark tradition. The book I've chosen to represent the entire century, however, is not a volume in which new discoveries were presented but one that has come to represent the acme of medical teaching. It had no effect on theory or on comprehension of the biological basis of healing. It was strictly instructional.

Given ten seconds to answer, how would any reader respond if asked to name a single medical textbook? Almost certainly, the reply would be, "Why, *Gray's Anatomy*, of course!" The answer would have been the same a century ago. Now in its thirty-ninth edition, this gradually revised workhorse of medical pedagogy has remained in everyday use far longer than any medical text of modern times, and it is likely to go on and on and on—as far as the futuristic eye can see. It outlives one after another of its editors, of whom the current work requires nineteen, with the addition of seventeen specialist contributors and an additional fifty international authorities to review specialized sections.

Yet the appearance of *Anatomy, Descriptive and Surgical* (the actual title of Henry Gray's classic) drew a harsh, derisive critique in *The Boston Medical and Surgical Journal*, as *The New England Journal of Medicine* was then called. The reviewer's scathing criticism took up fully half the journal's pages in two successive issues. Paragraph after paragraph described supposed errors and omissions. Of all the review's indictments, the most vehement was directed at Gray's illustrations. No doubt astonishing the medical students whose enthusiastic outpouring of pounds and dollars had made the book an immediate success, the reviewer disparaged the clarity of the drawings, their large number, even their very presence. To compound matters, he argued, Gray had chosen the worst possible course by labeling each structure in his pictures, rather than employing the footnoted numbers or letters customarily used by contemporary authors. That kind of pap made things too easy for medical students: clear, well-labeled diagrams would divert a young man's attention from a textbook's endless procession of sentences. "Let a student have general illustrations, and he will use them at the expense of the text," protested the reviewer. To the ascetic, puritan mind of the proper Bostonian, Gray's book looked like an illustrated road to pedagogical Hell.

But as other leading journals would note, that innovative way of presenting illustrations was one of the strengths of a book that also had many other praiseworthy qualities. In striking contrast to its rival American periodical, *The Lancet* ended a laudatory review with a line that remains as true in the twenty-first century as it was in 1858: "As a full, systematic, and advanced treatise on anatomy, combining the various merits of the volumes of many countries, scientifically excellent, and adapted to all the wants of the student, we are not acquainted with any work in any language, which can take equal rank with the one before us."

Who was the carping American critic, and what explains his fierce animosity toward a book whose advent was recognized by almost all other reviewers as a significant event in medical education—a book that elicited such an enthusiastic response from the students and practitioners for whom it was meant? The two-part screed is signed with the single letter *H*. That letter is as revealing as the *A* with which Nathaniel Hawthorne had startled American readers only a few years earlier. Gray's literary assassin was almost surely Harvard's professor of anatomy, Oliver Wendell Holmes, no mean scribbler himself. Who but Holmes would have been chosen to critique a major new textbook in his specialty for an important Boston journal? Who else would have been granted half the pages of two issues? And who else, rejecting the anonymity assumed by virtually all of the medical reviewers of his day, would have signed his work with a single initial, doubtless certain that his readers would easily identify him (and perhaps confident that the authority of his name would quash any objections to *his* objections)?

A clue to Holmes's motives may lie in a valedictory speech that the Autocrat of the Breakfast Table gave when he retired from the presidency of the Boston Medical Library in 1889. Holmes spoke of his reverence for a book familiarly known as "Sharpey and Quain," the foremost anatomy text of his teaching days. Holmes thought of that book, and two other anatomical tomes, as "the stepping stones of my professional life." His donation of those volumes to the library on that parting day "costs me a little heartache to take leave of such old and beloved companions." Could it be that the Autocrat's attack on the new textbook was motivated by his apprehension that it would displace his revered literary mainstay as *the* text for the instruction of medical students?

Gray's Anatomy would become a classic of pedagogical literature, one of the healing profession's truly great books. Dr. Holmes, ensconced on high among the immortals of American medicine, might be chagrined to find that the volume he so mercilessly maligned is familiar to all modern-day medical students, while the earthshaking works of Vesalius, Harvey, and Morgagni are barely, if at all, known to them. As for Sharpey and Quain, try the Internet.

GRIEF AND REFLECTION: AFTER 9/11

THIS ESSAY WAS WRITTEN ON SEPTEMBER 21, 2001, IN THE AFTERMATH
OF THE DESTRUCTION OF THE WORLD TRADE CENTER IN NEW YORK CITY.

Ten days later: faced with the anguish of so many who have been directly touched by our national tragedy, we seek means to unite ourselves with them. We scan the lengthening lists of those who have died and feel intense relief to find that we know not a single person; and yet something in us insistently whispers the tiniest sigh of regret that no familiar name appears. Psychiatrists are quoted in the papers about this troubling phenomenon, and they assuage our guilt by telling us that such thoughts have to do with our need to find solidarity with the dead and those who have loved them.

But we suspect that something else is afoot. We recognize it from our experience of funerals we have attended over the years. It is that small voice in each of us that expresses the hunger for belonging and even for some bit of validation by proclaiming, "*I, too*, am suffering—*I, too*, have been affected by this tragedy—Don't leave *me* out." Or perhaps only "*I* comprehend, *I* understand, *I* can feel the magnitude of this sadness." Joining in another's sorrow expresses, gratifies the insistent demands of that voice. This, too, may be a means of declaring solidarity. But perhaps it declares narcissism as well. So what?

Physicians whose specialties bring them into frequent contact with terminal patients and their circle of kith and kin are familiar with such feelings, because they are commonly manifested in the hours and days after a life has ended. We are familiar with other unwelcome emotions, too, whether they are the well-publicized survivors' guilt of people who have narrowly missed death or the schadenfreude about which we feel such shame when we recognize it in ourselves. These are patterns that for the most part affect only those who have had a close relationship with the dead. But we are now an entire nation of distant mourners, and the full range of human response is showing itself, though most of it is unspoken and even unacknowledged. In the coming sad months, many Americans will find themselves unprepared for their own (often conflicting) responses to the enormity of our nation's loss of life.

Grieving is an indescribably complex phenomenon. Even the grieving at a distance that most of us have been experiencing in these recent days is such a mix of cultural, experiential, and genetically determined variables in each individual that its totality eludes the most sensitive perceptions of the most sensitive observers, and sometimes of the most skilled too. Some responses that would seem reprehensible or aberrant are so common that they fall into the necessarily wide category called "normal." It is probably safe to say that only when symptoms are extreme, or refuse to ebb at a reasonable time, should they be considered pathological. Until that time—and who can with certainty declare its duration?—they are not in fact symptoms, for that word carries with it the connotation of sickness. And who is to say, beyond certain obviously bizarre behaviors, what is extreme? The group of professionals who deal with such matters would do well to avoid calling themselves "grief therapists." With only rare exceptions, they are not treating sick people. They are counselors or guides, not therapists, and I wish there were more of them. Then the varieties of mourning response might be more widely understood, and the mourners might be kinder to themselves.

We all know that mourning does recede, but far too few of us understand that it never ends. Certain stars disappear from our personal firmament once we have sustained a loss, no matter how remote that loss may be from the rhythm of our own daily concerns. Life resumes somewhat changed. When journalists and our leaders tell us in the immediate aftermath of the unutterable events of September 11 that our nation will never be the same, they are only stating a universal truth that applies to every loss in the life of every individual. But now, that truth is magnified by hundreds of millions who mourn, and it has become international in magnitude. Those who in the past have blathered about something they call "closure" must surely by now know that there is no such thing. We try to achieve a measure of acceptance to help us with the reality of loss, but even that is rarely complete. All of this must be taken into account in the calculus of what it means to be human.

In the first chapter of this book, I explained why I had chosen to call it—and in the process, call medicine too—"The Uncertain Art." After the most horrendous single catastrophe in our nation's history, few would deny that life itself is the source of our greatest uncertainty. Just as the philosophical underpinnings of medicine reflect the culture of the society it serves, the art of medicine reflects the reality of everything going on around it. Medicine is uncertain, life is uncertain, and the boundaries of grief are uncertain. We must allow grief to proceed as it will.

Ruminating on the less attractive features of our own grief is far more harmful to us than those features themselves. When we turn inward, it should be to reflect, not to be obsessed by guilt over the unwelcome thoughts that flow so readily into our minds. To become isolated in one's own sadness is to be deprived of the consolations that come with shared loss. Prayer services, wakes, shiva, communal vigils, the formalized nature of the funeral itself, the rituals and customs of the first period after a death—all these construct the edifice that society and organized religion have provided to enable us not only to express our sorrow but also to turn outward in order to do so.

Then there is the matter of carrying on. In the immediate aftermath of September 11, the airwaves were flooded with exhortations for us to return to normalcy as soon as possible. If we hesitated, we were told, the vicious perpetrators of this outrage against morality would achieve their objective. The smoothest path to recovery from grief was to be found in the minutiae and hurly-burly of daily life; restoring them should be our objective if we were to heal and if we were to frustrate the designs of those who would terrorize us into fear and inaction.

We were glad to hear such exhortations. When we return to the mundane without public sanction, it is too often with twinges of guilt for resuming our daily lives instead of lingering in sadness, out of loyalty to the dead and concern about the tragic events we have witnessed. Like good parents, the spokesmen for our culture's values urged us to face again the everyday challenges of our lives. Because they allowed us to turn in the direction to which our recuperating minds inclined, we did so less burdened by regret than we might otherwise have been.

In fact, we hardly needed such admonitions. Of course we would carry on. What else could we do? The human psyche will heal itself if the trauma is not repeatedly inflicted. It responds precisely the way injured flesh responds, and that includes the scar that is the constant reminder of what was endured. The scar tells us, among its other messages, that we are changed, both on the surface, where it is visible, and in deeper regions, where it is not. When we return to that familiar hurly-burly, we return with a new perspective. This, too, must be accepted. It is impossible to accept the loss completely; it is difficult to accept some of the unpalatable thoughts that assail us while mourning; but it is both easy and strengthening to accept the change that such a tragedy has wrought, especially if it makes us more self-aware and grateful for life, for the personal liberties we have heretofore taken for granted, and for the brotherhood of this great nation.

At this moment still so close to the hour of tragedy, we think of the months ahead and of how we will maintain the resolve, personal and national, that now comes so easily. Those of us who have been able to give little more than some money and some blood may, just by being reflective, be able to contribute something of consequence to the national good. Although we may applaud much of what we are hearing today of our government's planned response, a rush to action sometimes gets in the way of our taking the time to be with ourselves and to remember the eternal values that have sculpted the moral order and our nation. Our leaders will surely make errors in the coming months, but we can hope that they will not be errors of morality, even in their actions against those who quite obviously have none. As essential to the healing process as it is that we vent our individual and collective spleen against those who have declared us their satanic enemy; as therapeutic as it is that we cry out for justice and retribution and achieve them; as useful as it is that we dedicate ourselves to a resumption of normalcy so effective that it frustrates the purposes of the terror—as vital to healing, security, and the continuing triumph of liberty as such responses are, they will be of no enduring value unless we also, in our reflectiveness, address the inequities that have formed the background of such unbridled rage against the values that shape our democracy.

Religious freedom, individual liberty, and the unrestrained privilege of pursuing knowledge and commerce have made Western and Westernized nations the most prosperous, intellectually advanced, and healthy societies the world has ever known. And far greater advances are sure to come. The principles of democracy have brought benefits to the public health that were unimaginable a century ago. This is not true for those who are attempting to destroy our lives and our system of government. The misguided zealots who would bring us to our knees represent a philosophy meant to appeal to people left behind in the extraordinary advances of our time. Poverty, disease, constrained life expectancy, and utter lack of opportunity to affect their grim prospects have fostered the resentment that dismantles moral values, perverts religious doctrine, and fuels the flames with which the unenfranchised would immolate us. A self-righteous fury becomes the mood of an entire deprived culture, and its basis is despair. It is despair that is our enemy, not people.

Once we have dealt with the leaders who turn despair to their own ends, we must attend to the despair itself, and to the contempt for the value of human life from which it springs. We can best do that by treating it as we would treat an illness, for it is indeed a sickness of the soul. In an earlier chapter, I briefly mentioned the philosophy of the greatest pathologist of the nineteenth century, Rudolf Virchow of Berlin, who taught that disease is the product of the societal conditions in which it arises, namely poverty, ignorance, and the inattention of the affluent to the problems of the disadvantaged. A hundred years earlier, Pierre Cabanis, the eminent French medical philosopher, had written, "Sickness is dependent on the blunders of society," and called upon governments to redress the wrongs. Virchow took up the cause and urged his colleagues to change the conditions that breed sickness and unrest. "Physicians are the natural attorneys of the poor," he thundered, but his words were heeded by only a few. It is ironic that we have long recognized that the crime and misery of our inner cities are largely the result of inequality of opportunity, but we seem not to make the analogy with entire cultures. Nothing in the teachings of Islam stands in the way of the prosperity and scientific uplifting of its adherents; witness the extraordinary accomplishments of its civilization in the centuries after it exploded out of the Arabian Peninsula.

Whether they perceive it or not, the Islamic fundamentalists and those who share their desperation hate us far less for what *we* are than for what *they* are. In our own self-righteousness, we should not ignore the sources of theirs. Insofar as the industrialized nations can rally together to do it, we must fulfill a neglected obligation: it is now incumbent on us as never before to recognize that we are fighting a form of disease. Answering Rudolf Virchow's call, we must become physicians to the world. Every group—whatever its religious beliefs—left behind by the benisons of the past century should become our patient.

But there is another principle of disease and healing that must not be forgotten if our quest is to be successful, and it was articulated long before the philosophies of Cabanis and Virchow. Except when dealing with nations whose value systems we consider on a level with our own—the Marshall Plan is a case in point—Americans helping to build or rebuild another nation have too often been guilty of what so many of our critics justifiably call "cultural imperialism." Our intent should be to address sickness, poverty, and despair by giving direct aid and by teaching populations to be self-sufficient and to take advantage of present-day science, agriculture, and commerce. The point is not to make little Americas of them. Even the preaching of democracy should not be one of our goals. The very old principle of healing to which I refer was first articulated in the corpus of writings long attributed to Hippocrates. The author of Book I of *Epidemics* enjoins physicians in a declaration often misquoted in Latin as *primum non nocere* but which is best translated from the original Greek simply as "do no harm." The harm of cultural imperialism has been incalculable, not only to nations exposed to it but to ourselves as well. It is bad enough in the eyes of the bereft that we are privileged without seeming to deserve our good fortune; but to parade arrogance about our values is an outrage.

Let us recognize and address the needs of the sufferers in other lands and lessen the sum of human despair. Perhaps this is among the ways in which we can best express solidarity with those many adults and children whose loved ones were taken from them by the atrocities of September 11. Perhaps this is among the ways that we can honor the dead. It will not be sufficient to bring justice to their murderers or practical reparations to their survivors. We must do far more. We can add to the meaning of their lives by adding to the meaning of their deaths, if we turn our grief to reflection and our mourning to a search for paths toward peace and security for all the peoples of the world.

LIGHTNING ON MY MIND

Plus ça change, plus c'est la même chose.

Or perhaps not. Some things do change, and in unexpected ways. Even though I'd prepared myself for what I was going to see that morning, it was still disturbing to come face-to-face with it. All four patients were sitting dull and motionless on a long bench backed against the far wall of the psychiatric clinic's holding area, oblivious to one another's presence and to anyone else's. I hadn't expected them to notice me entering, but they also seemed totally unaware of the two chattering middle-aged nurses a-bustle within a few feet of them, riffling through charts, unlocking medication cabinets, laying out syringes and intravenous tubing—doing all the little jobs of starting up the early-morning activities of an outpatient clinic in a large urban hospital.

Three of the bench's occupants were women, one in each decade of life from the late thirties to near sixty. The older two were frumpily dressed in unpressed housecoats and worn sneakers. But the third woman wore a neat skirt and blouse and good shoes with a bit of heel. She had carefully combed her long black hair, though the total effect was only to add pallor to her wan, expressionless face. Sitting there with her body pressed against the arm of the bench, she might have been the melancholy wife of the gaunt, fortyish man slouching on the opposite end, separated from her by the older two and an impenetrable gulf of silence. She was no one's wife, however. Like the other three, she was a severely depressed outpatient, awaiting an electroshock treatment.

Of course, the four were not nearly as unresponsive as they appeared. There was in fact a firestorm going on in their brains, but none of it was directed to anything outside their own heads. Totally internal and only partly conscious, this firestorm left no energy for visible emotion or any but the most essential movements. All the people on that bench were embroiled in their own private wars; they were battling mental chaos, fear, and the relentless taunting of silent accusers denouncing them as worthless.

I have spoken to many severely depressed men and women, and all of them tell me similar things. During the worst of their illness, they are too fully absorbed in the struggle with their clamoring demons to have anything left for the world. They are without strength or resilience. What is far worse, they are without hope. The leaden heaviness of hearts burdened with the loss of a future and the belittling of a past bows their heads and bends their backs. The forlorn sight I witnessed that morning was the face of despair. Yet all of this is almost always supposed to be cured, miraculously, by a few jolts of electricity to the brain. The undeniable—and largely unexplainable—clinical result of electroshock therapy is that the symptoms of a great majority of deeply depressed patients disappear entirely following a series of treatments, usually not exceeding six or eight. No one has yet been able to figure out the precise mechanism by which this peculiar form of therapy does its astonishing work.

As early as the sixteenth century, the Swiss medical innovator Paracelsus was treating lunacy by inducing convulsions with oral doses of tincture of camphor. Over the years, many other doctors followed suit, attempting to shock people out of their symptoms. Because there were some successes, the methods persisted throughout that long period when efficacy was far more important than explanation. Then, in the 1930s, a group of Italian psychiatrists observed that some of their epileptic patients who were also depressed became free of their mental symptoms when they went through a period of particularly frequent convulsions. Concluding that there is some biological incompatibility between seizures and mental illness, the psychiatrists began looking for a patient so seriously psychotic that a failed experiment in electrically induced fits could not possibly worsen his condition. But first they had to satisfy themselves that the current they planned to use for the induction of the seizures would not be lethal. This they did by paying a visit to a Rome slaughterhouse where pigs were dispatched after being rendered unconscious with a standard current. None of the animals succumbed to the electricity, and the researchers were encouraged to seek out an appropriate human subject.

Their opportunity came one day in April 1938, when the police brought in a disheveled and unidentifiable thirty-nine-year-old man who had been found wandering through the Rome railway station, mumbling and sometimes shouting gibberish. The rest of the story, as described by an eyewitness, is worth recording for posterity. After observing the potential patient for a fortnight, the physicians decided that he fit the criteria for their ideal candidate. They began their human experiment with some trepidation, administering a dose of only 70 volts of current for two-tenths of a second. Even that small amount threw their subject into a brief grand mal seizure. After the final spasm, he forced his head upward against the restraints that held him, and shouted angrily and obscenely, *"Che cazzo fai!"* This was the first lucid sentence he had uttered since being brought to the hospital. The doctors were initially worried by the force of the convulsive response—both the physical and the verbal part—but, relieved that they had not killed their subject, they eventually felt justified in raising the current to 110 volts for half a second. After a single jolt, the patient immediately became well oriented to his surroundings and began speaking sensibly, sans obscenities. After ten more treatments he seemed fully cured. Later on he suffered a relapse, but the doctors were nevertheless elated at the outcome of their experiment, since even a temporary improvement held the promise of more enduring relief for patients less sick. The Italians and numerous other psychiatrists were able to confirm the salubrious results in other patients, many of whom remained well. So-called electroconvulsive therapy, or ECT, became the rage. It was thought that the current somehow modified thinking patterns, or perhaps obliterated pathological memories; but the biochemical basis of the treatment's success remained a mystery.

Nowadays it is known that a cascade of neurotransmitters—with names like serotonin, dopamine, norepinephrine, and the like—is released into the brain's circulation at the time of the shock. How this might have a lasting effect on mental functioning is still undetermined. The one certainty is that electroshock therapy usually does what is expected of it. After decades in which, for a variety of reasons, the therapy fell into disuse and even disrepute, it is again being widely utilized in the treatment of various forms of depression, both neurotic and psychotic, that do not respond to medications or a reasonable period of psychotherapy. The results have been remarkably good. The four people I saw sitting on the outpatient bench were staking their futures on that promise.

It was time to start work. One of the two nurses lightly touched the arm of the younger woman. She rose slowly, managing a small smile as though finally sensing that she was not alone in the holding area. Nurse and patient walked wordlessly into the adjoining room, where an anesthesiologist had just set up his equipment. Beside him stood the psychiatrist, a cheerful and very attractive woman about the same age as the patient. She took a step forward, and the two hugged warmly, as though they were close friends. And friendship, in fact, is precisely the right term for the relationship that had developed between them. The patient was about to undergo her fourth treatment and was showing enough improvement to begin paying attention to her appearance once more. In the loosening grip of pathological apathy, she had on her last visit asked the psychiatrist for advice about grooming. They were now sisters of a sort, and there was genuine tenderness in their embrace.

But the scrub-suited anesthesiologist was new to the young woman, and he introduced himself as she wearily drew her thin, taut body onto the gurney. After he had inserted an intravenous line into her left forearm, the psychiatrist gently affixed a wired electrode to each temple, having first taken care to smear it generously with conductive jelly to avoid burning at the points of contact with the skin. Electroencephalographic monitoring leads were then placed on the forehead, and one of the nurses attached the electrocardiogram and a blood pressure apparatus. The members of the medical team kept up a steady stream of small talk to distract their patient.

When everything was in place, the anesthesiologist injected a dose of Brevital (a barbiturate so named because it acts with great brevity) into the intravenous line, followed by the muscle relaxant Anectine, to induce a virtual paralysis of the entire body. The patient promptly fell into a comalike sleep. A bite block was now inserted between the woman's teeth to avoid any possibility that she might clamp down on her tongue during the ECT. After filling his patient's lungs with an extra load of oxygen to sustain her during an anticipated brief period of respiratory arrest, the anesthesiologist nodded to the others.

All was now ready. The psychiatrist pressed a button on the complex multidialed console controlling the electrical charge to be delivered, and the current coursed into the sleeping woman's brain. It passed from one temple to the other for a period of twenty-five seconds. I watched carefully for any evidence of convulsive activity or muscle spasm, but all I saw was a sudden upward turning and then twitching of the feet. Had I not been paying attention to the encephalogram and cardiogram, I would hardly have known that anything unusual was going on inside the patient's still body.

I was momentarily alarmed to see that the woman's heart abruptly arrested for a period of two seconds as the current began streaming through her brain. But it gradually resumed its normal rhythm within no more than ten beats, although her blood pressure—which had leaped to 240/120—stayed high the entire time. From their previous normally symmetric appearance, the brain waves being recorded on the electroencephalogram took on a spindly shape recognizable as the pattern of a seizure. This was sustained as long as the current flowed. But other than the spasmodic movements of the feet, there was no convulsion.

As the treatment drew to a close, the spasm of the feet turned into a brief series of rhythmic jerks, but that was the only visible evidence that one hundred joules of electricity had traveled through the woman's brain. In all other ways, she looked at this point like any healthy patient undergoing anesthesia for a minor surgical procedure. She awoke, was helped from the table, and seemed fully aware of her surroundings.

Having assured the doctors that she felt well, the patient was escorted to the corridor, where a friend was waiting to take her home. Scarcely ten minutes had elapsed since she was called from her place on the bench. She had not been required to change into a hospital gown. To judge from the way she looked, she might have just arisen from a short nap on the gurney—a power nap, so to speak.

The other patients, in turn, were led into the room and given their treatments. All responded just as the younger woman had. Checking the large clock on the wall, I noted that completing all four of the treatments had taken less than an hour. I was told that the patients might experience a period of amnesia covering the fifteen or twenty minutes before and after the session, but otherwise no mental aberrations were to be expected. It was as simple as that. After more sessions like this—perhaps as few as three or four—the patient would become all that she or he had been before depression stole the real world away. The psychiatrist told me of one patient who had gone to his law office and worked on briefs after his fourth and fifth treatments. His early-morning visits to the clinic were only short interruptions of his gradually normalizing day.

How different all this was from the first time that I, as a third-year medical student in 1953, saw a patient undergoing ECT. She was confined to a huge state hospital, and few even marginally effective psychotropic drugs were available then; electroconvulsive therapy played a major role in the treatment of the seriously ill. In those days, the onset of convulsion was a moment of high drama and some danger, because there were no muscle relaxants to prevent the massive seizures induced by unmodulated electroshock.

On that morning more than half a century ago, some twenty patients were assembled in a dingy, poorly lit hallway lined with parallel wooden benches. Those not bundled in robes and pajamas were wearing drab, ill-fitting clothing. All but two or three of the men were unshaven and uncombed. Most of the women appeared considerably older than the age given on their hospital charts. Even the youngest among them—two girls in their late teens—looked as if they had just stepped out of a Walker Evans photograph of the joyless wives of Alabama sharecroppers.

Though some of the patients were far enough along in their treatment to display real interest in their surroundings, most were as uncommunicative and dispirited as the people I would see in the outpatient clinic so many years later. As their names were called, they were taken into a small adjoining room, where a short, heavyset man with a thick Hispanic accent awaited them, accompanied by six powerfully built young attendants dressed in rumpled white uniforms. The routine on the morning I visited hadn't changed since its introduction into the hospital shortly after the great Italian successes—though it would begin to alter with the development of muscle relaxants only a few years later. The heavy door of the soundproof chamber would be slammed shut, and one of the muscular young men would guide the patient into a supine position on the narrow treatment table. When I entered with the middle-aged woman I had been following on the ward, I realized that the older man with the accent was the psychiatrist who was to administer both the anesthetic and the ECT. Considering the grim surroundings, he spoke to his patient with surprising gentleness as he inserted the IV for the first of what would be a series of perhaps ten treatments. But she barely responded to his words or to the prick of the needle piercing her pale skin. Even when the young aides surrounded her and applied thick leather restraints to her extremities and waist, she lay perfectly still. After injecting the drug to put her to sleep, the psychiatrist placed a wired electrode on each temple, but there was no electrocardiogram, no electroencephalogram, and no monitoring of vital signs—only a mouth block, which was merely a tongue depressor wrapped in layers of tape.

The electrode wires led to a small wooden box, perhaps four by six inches in size, plugged directly into a wall outlet—the source of the unmodified 110-volt current to be used. Having turned the box's control dial to the setting marked "medium" (the other choices were "high" and "low"), the psychiatrist then delivered a powerful blast of electricity that threw the patient into massive convulsions of every muscle in her body, resembling an extreme form of grand mal epileptic seizure in which head, arms, and legs strained repeatedly upward against the leather straps and the strong hands of the six orderlies holding the patient down. In spite of their strenuous attempts to prevent it, she seemed about to leap upward off the table with every jolting thrust of her trunk. Her face turned blue with the effort; foamy spittle dribbled from the corners of her mouth, while her body spasmodically attempted to jerk itself double at the waist restraint, like a long, thin jackknife trying to snap shut over and over again. To a twenty-two-year-old medical student, it was a horrible sight.

Though the table was padded, it was not unknown for the violent thrashing about to result in crushed vertebrae or fractured extremities. Since elderly people with fragile bones were especially prone to such serious complications, the doctors were reluctant to treat them. As a consequence, the hospital's wards were full of aging, severely depressed men and women who passed their last years in abject desolation because nothing could be done for them.

My patient awakened slowly. Dazed, confused, and glassy-eyed, she had no idea where or even who she might be. After a few minutes, I helped her up—wobbly as she still was—and clumsily half-walked, half-dragged her past the forlorn group waiting outside. I then took her back to the ward in a wheelchair. Within a short time she fell into a deep sleep, lasting about three hours, and awoke amnesic for everything that had occurred in her entire life. By the late afternoon, most— but far from all—of her memory had returned. In two or three days she would be taken back for another treatment. Each time, the unrecoverable part of her memory loss grew greater; each time, her depression lessened. ECT was a difficult and dangerous form of therapy in those days, but despite its devastating side effects, it worked.

It works better today, as I witnessed on that morning in the outpatient clinic. Electroshock therapy is in the midst of a renaissance, but its associations with the grim scenes of yesteryear still linger. It is time for the fear to be dispersed; we are not dealing with *la même chose*. Having returned in twenty-first-century clothing, ECT has taken its place among the growing number of biomedical wonders. No longer to be viewed as a last resort or dreaded as an agent of psychic destruction, it is truly a modern miracle.

SCATOLOGICAL MEDICINE

Who remembers Serutan? In ads that began to appear about seventy-five years ago on billboards and public transportation and in the pages of periodicals, it was touted as "Nature's Aid to Elimination!" The very name of the anticonstipation medicine was "Nature's" spelled backward, a disclosure made in the text of every ad. As a boy who frequently rode the New York subways in the 1930s and 1940s, I used to wonder what physiological failure awaited me a few decades hence that would require a patent remedy described as having been developed specifically for use "after 35." At the age of nine or ten, I tried to guess which of the dour commuters sitting near me had failed to take their Serutan that morning.

Serutan has long since been replaced by a wide variety of agents that range from those "recommended by your doctor," like Metamucil, to the botanical therapies found in health food stores. Though Americans are not as bowel-obsessed as some nationalities (think, for example, of the English), our annual consumption of stool softeners, laxatives, and similar propellants is enormous. In this, we differ little from the Sumerians. In the medical annals of every civilization that has left sufficient records, there is some mention of the need to keep the bowels open. Worship at the shrine of the god called Regularity is common. Its worldwide congregation exceeds in size the total number of people attending church, synagogue, and mosque services on any given weekend; it is a faith whose scripture grows ever larger.

Before humankind discovered the earliest rudiments of science, medical symptoms were commonly attributed to supernatural causes: the gods were angry and manifested their displeasure by bringing disease. It has been much the same with Regularity. If the god called Regularity feels that insufficient or derogatory attention has been paid to him, he sickens the sinner with headache, lassitude, nausea, nervousness, and impotence—some of the symptoms that early cultures ascribed to constipation. In more sophisticated times, such complex pathologies as tuberculosis, gallstones, and cancer have been added to the list.

Of all the ancient peoples, the Egyptians seem to have been most attentive to the commandments of Regularity. Papyri depict a culture permeated with a rectal mythology that influenced day-to-day behavior and supported the equivalent of an industry. The putrefied effluvium of fecal matter, called *wehuduw*, was said to be absorbed through the bowel wall into a system of ducts that under ordinary circumstances carried a healthful mixture of air, water, and blood outward from the heart to the other organs of the body. Once in the vessels, the contaminant forced its way back to the heart and from there was driven centrifugally to poison every tissue. The various measures used to prevent the accumulation of wehuduw apparently became less effective as one grew older, so that many of the symptoms nowadays associated with aging were thought to be caused by its malign influence. Elderly Egyptians were believed to die of constipation as we now do of arteriosclerosis. Wehuduw was the cholesterol of its time.

And what were the preventive measures? They appear to have been little different from the ones employed by many of today's worshipers of Regularity. On three consecutive days each month, every person took a cathartic prophylactically. If more coprodynamism was needed (and very likely even if it was not), enemas were administered. In fact, the best available evidence indicates that enemas were invented by the Egyptians, for the express purpose of preventing accumulation of wehuduw. Care of the rectum became a medical specialty, personified in the form of a physician known as the Shepherd of the Anus, a particularly elevated designation in the hierarchy of Egyptian healing. His job was to guide members of the privileged classes, including the pharaoh, through the process of effective elimination and to give enemas when indicated. He was Regularity's high priest. Among his methods was the anal instillation of honey under pressure, which was believed to neutralize the toxic products in the stool. Cease wondering about the enigmatic face of the Sphinx—it is doubtless the ambivalent response to a rectum packed tightly with the sweet golden nectar of the bee.

With the advent of Greek medicine, the doctrine of the four humors gave further sanction to the use of therapeutic intestinal cleansers. Though the toxic effects of feces continued to rank high among the theoretical causes of symptoms, it was actually the surfeit of the humors that most concerned the doctors. Powerful laxatives were among the treatments thought most effective against excesses of yellow and black bile, which were supposed to cause many illnesses.

But with or without humoral explanations for disease, a good cleanout remained, until fairly recently, an important treatment used by healers or as a home remedy. By the late seventeenth century, every sophisticated Frenchman considered the enema an essential part of his daily toilet. Many of the botanicals that were a mainstay of both the physician's pharmacopoeia and the home medicine box as recently as a century ago functioned as purgatives or emetics. Medical and kitchen table dogma demanded that the poisons be disgorged in one direction or the other.

Like most of the medical and lay attacks on disease, the use of purges and pukes had no scientific basis. Though real science began to affect medicine in the seventeenth century, two more centuries would pass before the old notions of therapy were replaced by methods based on experimental studies verifiable in laboratories. And then, paradoxically, the very evidence that should have given the lie to the efficacy of internal purity came to be used as a justification for ever more vigorous efforts to sustain its importance in the doctor's quiver of therapeutic arrows.

In 1867, Joseph Lister reported his observation that infection in postsurgical wounds was the result of contamination with certain bacteria similar to those that Louis Pasteur, a decade earlier, had shown to be the cause of putrefaction in the wine and beer produced by distillers near Lille. The next several decades brought a series of discoveries that became the basis of the germ theory of disease. Sicknesses previously thought to be the result of bad air, bad morals, atmospheric events, constitutional weakness, or even the not-quite-discarded humoral imbalances were shown in fact to be caused by infestation with organisms invisible to the naked eye. These organisms lived in "the world of the infinitely small," as Pasteur called the realm revealed by the microscope. The elaboration of germ theory revolutionized medical thinking, determined the direction of research for the next century, and provided straightforward explanations for phenomena that doctors and grandmothers had been talking about for millennia. Among them was the profession's certainty—and the laity's, too—that constipated people are prone to develop debilitating symptoms and even diseases.

The scientifically minded physician—alert to the latest findings of the research laboratories—at last had an explanation for the pernicious power of a stalled stool. The bacteria seen swarming in the decomposing feces were doubtless releasing a powerful poison into the circulatory system. And there was another factor, from the emerging field of physiological chemistry: the demonstration that the breakdown of proteins in the feces released compounds that were often toxic. After thousands of years of vagueness, the problem had been solved: bacteria and noxious organic compounds were the culprits. This convincing proposition was dubbed with a resplendent name that reflected the specialized knowledge its discoverers had brought to bear in tracking it down. Poisoning by one's own retained or reluctant stool was henceforth to be known as "autointoxication," so designated by a French physician and biologist named Charles Bouchard. To establish his priority in the field of posteriority, Bouchard wrote an influential book about it in 1887, *Lectures in Autointoxication.*

Over the next half century, a wide variety of methods—scientific, quasi-scientific, pseudoscientific, and downright phony—appeared, intended to relieve the scourge of feckless feces. Some of the names associated with the constipation crusades became household words: John Harvey Kellogg of Battle Creek, Michigan, who championed vegetarianism, corn flakes, and colonic irrigation and offered free treatment at his sanitarium to those who were unfortunate enough to be simultaneously bloated and impecunious; Élie Metchnikoff, a Nobel Prize winner for his discovery of phagocytosis, who promoted the consumption of yogurt to restore the proper bacterial mix in the intestine; Bernarr Macfadden, who became famous for adding the bulky diet to his advocacy of strenuous physical therapy for vibrant health; and Charles Atlas, who decried the clogging of the anatomical area he called the "internal sewer" and insisted that his acolytes take prunes, figs, and three or four "internal baths" during their twelve-week muscle-building correspondence course. "What would you think of a fireman," his instructional literature demanded, "who continually choked up his furnace with coal and never cleared out the accumulated ash?"

But two stars shine with particular luminosity in the scatological sky. One was ultimately proved to be a fraud and a huckster, though it must be said that he did sincerely believe in the notion of fecal poisoning. The other was one of the leading surgeons of England, convinced that the battle against autointoxication was to be fought on scientific grounds and won in the operating room.

First, the huckster. On his arrival in New York from his native England around 1880, Charles Tyrell was hospitalized for the treatment of an otherwise unspecified paralysis. While being treated—unsuccessfully—he read a tract by a certain A. Wilford Hall, Ph.D., advancing the thesis that every disease can be cured or prevented by frequent flushings of the colon. Tyrell followed Hall's written advice and was soon healthy. A few years later, he established a business called the Hygienic Institute and wrote a book about his newfound catholicon, *The Royal Road to Health*. The book was widely read, as were several pamphlets on the same subject; they urged patients to purchase, for $12.50, a colonic cleansing device invented by the author: the J.B.L. (for Joy, Beauty, Life) Cascade, which was to be used to administer a warm mixture of fluids (contents undisclosed) three or four times each week.

The new product was immediately successful. Testimonials poured in from all over North America and several foreign countries. Tyrell happily used them in his widespread advertising; business boomed, and people began buying the Cascade as a gift for friends, business associates, and even brides. Successive editions of *The Royal Road to Health* sold as well as the enema devices, and more than a hundred printings were necessary to satisfy the demand. A scientific gloss was put on the book after 1907, when Metchnikoff published his acclaimed book *The Prolongation of Life*. Without consulting the great scientist, Tyrell used some of the book's arguments about the salubrious qualities of yogurt to bolster his statements about the importance of colonic cleanliness.

All of this was going on at a time when medical fraud was rampant in the United States. In response to the growing problem, the American Medical Association established a department that came to be called the Bureau of Investigation. The bureau soon began looking into the safety of the Cascade. Under the direction of its chief—the appropriately named Dr. Arthur J. Cramp—the bureau's investigations disclosed that Tyrell, a former actor who referred to himself as "Doctor," had obtained his MD degree only in 1900, when he was fifty-seven years old, from a short-lived New York school called the Eclectic Institute. Though he had often stated that Mother Nature needed nothing more than pure water to clean out the intestines, his mysterious solution contained borax (a harsh chemical that can injure the intestine) and salt. A number of other questionable facts turned up as well, prompting *The Journal of the American Medical Association* to publish a statement warning customers about the product. Many of those who stopped the irrigations in response to the article were shocked to discover that their colonic function was no longer spontaneous and would recover slowly, if at all. But the AMA had no power to punish Tyrell, and more than a few of the suckers born every minute continued to use his product until the theory of autointoxication was definitively disproved in the early 1920s, a few years after Tyrell's death as a rich man.

William Arbuthnot Lane, surgeon to London's Guy's Hospital, was another case entirely. Lane was convinced that man's assumption of the upright position had resulted in the unnatural descent of the abdominal organs into positions in which they hung by their own weight, putting stress on the ligaments and other tissues from which they had once been suspended without tension, and causing angularities. The stagnant passage of food and stool, slowed down by these so-called

Lane's kinks, allowed the autointoxicants to be absorbed into the bloodstream. An additional factor in Lane's thinking was a concept then becoming current as a result of the rapidly evolving germ theory. In their inexperience at interpreting microscopic observations, most physicians believed that the intestinal tract's normal state was sterility and that it contributed nothing to digestion. Therefore, they thought that the vast bacterial colonization of the colon was a pathological condition. To Lane, this meant that the theory of fecal stasis had been put on an up-to-date clinical footing. By 1903, he began to excise surgically all or a large portion of the colons of patients referred to him for the treatment of the many illnesses said to result from autointoxication—diabetes, rheumatoid arthritis, gastric ulcer, thyroid disease, and epilepsy among them. In the following year, his judgment was substantiated by a meeting with Metchnikoff, who would later write, in *The Nature of Man*: "It is no longer rash to say that not only the rudimentary appendage [appendix] but the whole of the large in-testine [is] superfluous, and that their removal would be attended with happy results." Similar previous statements by other authorities had influenced George Bernard Shaw to write *The Doctor's Dilemma* in 1906.

Lane became a zealot for his cause, undeterred (pun unavoidable) by the questionable therapeutic outcomes—not to mention the 24 percent mortality rate in his thousands of operated cases. He was made a baronet in 1913 and, as Sir Arbuthnot, became one of the wealthiest surgeons in the world.

Ironically, this was the same year in which the skeptics were begin-ning to provide strong evidence against the notions on which his operation was founded. During the next two decades the theory was battered on all sides—by radiologic, biochemical, clinical, and micro-scopic studies—and finally debunked. There has never been any sus-tainable evidence that absorption of toxic products from the lower bowel causes a single one of the symptoms or diseases that have so long been attributed to it. The headache, lassitude, and general sense of ill-being that do in fact occur in obstinate constipation have been shown to be the result of mechanical distension and irritation of the rectum by impacted masses of stool. There is no such thing as auto-intoxication.

But to call it a passing (oh, dear—another of those insistent puns) fad would not be entirely correct. The notion of autointoxication was based on an inextinguishable myth, namely the existence of the god Regularity. Though science disproved his existence, few of the faithful stopped believing. Whether overtly or in secret, the convinced still worship. Would that they might harken to the words of one of Arbuthnot Lane's leading opponents, Sir Arthur Hurst, who in 1935 wrote what he thought would be an epitaph for feces fixation:

> The vast army of hypochondriacs, who are never happy unless their stools conform to an ideal which they have invented for themselves, can only be cured by making themselves realize that feces have no standard size, shape, consistence nor color; they are then ready to follow the example of the dog rather than that of the cat—and never look behind them.

HIPPOCRATES REDUX

On June 24, 1889, a youth of twenty—forever after to be memorialized in the literature of medicine by his initials, G.H.—was punitively discharged from the Johns Hopkins Hospital eight days after an operation. Only the second patient to have undergone a newly devised method of hernia repair, he had been found guilty of "insubordination." His offense? In the words by which he is fated to be remembered for as long as medical historians study the origins of modern surgical techniques, "Patient got out of bed several times and took cathartic pills without permission." The punishment decreed by the surgeon, William Halsted, was nothing compared with that meted out by the young man's seemingly taxed tissues. Three years later, the repentant G.H. returned to the hospital with a palpable loop of squishy bowel in his scrotum, signifying "a complete return of the hernia." Of the first ten patients followed for a period sufficient to test the effectiveness of the new technique, G.H. was the only one to develop a recurrence; he was also the only one to get out of bed before the prescribed three weeks. To the surgeons of the time, it was QED: Get out of bed too early, and your stitches will not hold.

Young G.H. was one of the astonishingly high number of patients who don't follow doctors' orders. In Halsted's time, their sin was called "insubordination"; fifty years later, it was "recalcitrance"; today the preferred term is "noncompliance" or, if one is striving to avoid any connotation of medical paternalism, "nonadherence." No one is sure just how many noncompliant patients there are, but in the studies of prescribed medications that serve as a rough index of such things, the figure averages 50 percent; in one survey, of cases in which children depended on a parent to administer oral penicillin, the rate was 92 percent. At least one-third of hospital admissions for heart failure are necessitated by neglect of dietary or pharmacologic instructions. Many of these patients are elderly, and their noncompliance is caused by such factors as forgetfulness, confusion, cost, intolerance of minor side effects, lack of a social support system, and, finally, complacency after having been relieved of their symptoms by the very therapy that they therefore abandon.

Not all patients end up in the kind of jam in which G.H. found himself. The reasons why some (though not many) get away with medical self-neglect are uncertain, but one of them is surely that in some cases the treatment was not necessary in the first place. We physicians have been taught to categorize our patients and deal with their illnesses by following the algorithm that certain findings should necessarily lead to certain treatments. In the vast majority of cases this approach is appropriate and effective, but sometimes it is found wanting because we have not considered individual variations. The same disease may have different manifestations in different ways in different patients, and therapy should be modified accordingly.

And even a noncomplier's relapse or therapeutic unresponsiveness cannot necessarily be ascribed to his failure to follow instructions; there may be other reasons for the poor result. G.H., in fact, is the perfect example. With today's knowledge of wound healing, we can be sure that he could not have done himself harm by getting out of bed and swallowing a few cathartic pills eight full days after a technically adequate hernia repair. In his case, "subsequent" does not equal "consequent." The fact is that Halsted's new technique was not perfect. It is also quite possible that the surgeon (who was later disclosed to be secretly addicted first to cocaine and then to morphine) was not in good form on the day of operation. The recurrence of hernia almost certainly had nothing to do with G.H.'s felony. Halsted's new method was a significant improvement over previous ones, but it was hardly surefire. In his early cases, there were seven recurrences among the fifty-three compliant patients who had been studied long enough, a relapse rate of approximately 13 percent even when all instructions were obeyed. Of course, none of this contradicts the obvious fact that, for almost everyone, the best way to overcome disease or disability is to find a good doctor and do what he or she says. Today's recurrence rate for first-time hernia repair in compliant patients is under 3 percent.

All this is a way of leading myself back to the First Aphorism of Hippocrates. Recall that the second chapter of this book was devoted to a parsing of the first sentence of that ancient maxim. Recollect also that I promised (or threatened) to get back to the second sentence at a later point. That point has now been reached. Here is the entire aphorism, circa 300 B.C.E., translated from its Greek original:

> Life is short, and the Art is long; the occasion fleeting; experience fallacious, and judgment difficult. The physician must not only be prepared to do what is right himself, but also to make the patient, the attendants, and the externals, cooperate.

The crucial element in the patient's cooperation would seem to be compliance, about which there are some hard-to-erase myths. One is that socioeconomically advantaged people are unlikely to stray from a prescribed therapeutic plan. In fact, one study after another has shown the opposite to be true: nonadherence is so widespread among all social, ethnic, and otherwise categorizable groups that it cannot be predicted based on the characteristics of patients. Inattention to such findings can result in some dangerous misjudgments, not only in the management of individuals but in the equitable treatment of entire populations. For example, some clinicians have considered it appropriate to withhold HIV triple-drug therapy from patients with serious personal or social problems, on the assumption that they are likely to abandon treatment and thereby become a reservoir of drug-resistant strains. Not only is this a violation of patients' rights, but it forestalls the possibility of invoking any strategy for enhancing the reliability of the infected individuals. Compliance is improved by involving patients in the design of individualized treatment plans that suit their distinctive circumstances and by providing support and even incentives when enthusiasm flags. It does not help to stigmatize either the individuals who have lapsed or the groups who have been deemed least trust-worthy. Treating noncompliant people as though they are guilty of aberrant behavior not only reveals ignorance of the problem's high fre-quency across the board but alienates those who most need encourage-ment. Avoiding such criticism falls under the Hippocratic aphorism's admonition that the doctor must be "prepared to do what is right him-self," a goal he can accomplish only by making the patient a partner in his own management. But the patient's cooperation is not limited to compliance, nor is it even limited to situations in which disease has al-ready appeared. We know a great deal nowadays about the behaviors that are likely to maintain good health, prevent specific diseases, de-crease the probability of injury, and slow down the inevitable wear and tear of the aging process. Almost all of us are aware that we should avoid unhealthful foods and add healthful ones to our diets; get plenty of exercise; practice safe sex; stay away from certain drugs; refrain from smoking; stay out of direct sun as much as possible; be temperate with alcohol; check our bodies for lumps, bumps, sores, changing moles, and unusual or altered secretions; maintain a normal weight; wear seat belts and bicycle helmets; and observe certain precautions when traveling to foreign countries. Contrary to the Hippocratic in-junction, a doctor cannot be expected to "make" us cooperate in these matters. When we follow the well-known guidelines, we say that we are taking responsibility for our own health.

But does this mean that a chronic sunbather, a couch potato, or a fatty is irresponsible? Despite the temptation, answering "yes" is tan-tamount to making a moral judgment. Is it fair to blame the patient for acquiring certain diseases, as so many of the self-righteous have re-cently taken to doing? Considering the costs and social consequences of poor health, am I a bad citizen if I reach for a second helping of dessert or let my gym membership lapse? The fact is that many of us are critical of the obese and get angry if someone smokes in our vicin-ity, an anger not really justified by the danger that such a minimal single exposure poses to our own health. Our criticism and anger are likely to be intermingled with a touch of contempt, as though we slen-der abstainers were somehow better than the rule breakers. When they get sick, we say they have "brought it on themselves," and we wonder, sometimes aloud and even with the intent of influencing policy, why we should be paying their bills with our insurance premiums and taxes. This could not have been what the followers of Hippocrates had in mind. The reward for taking good care of oneself is the probability of improved health, not the attainment of moral superiority.

Anyway, how far should personal responsibility go? The media nowadays exhort us to identify the hospitals with the best record of treating the disease for which we are seeking care; check the credentials of our physicians and ask them about their level of experience; become familiar with the various sources of health information on the Internet; prepare a list of questions when we visit a doctor and make notes of the answers; and, if hospitalized, learn all the precautions that must be followed to minimize the many "nosocomial errors" (hospital-acquired health problems) so frequently reported on the evening news. The medical institution whose patient divisions, laboratories, and operating rooms I have prowled for half a century now provides a brochure titled "Patient Safety: Staying Safe in the Hospital," whose aim is to help patients protect themselves against what the introductory paragraph calls "unfortunate occurrences." "Do not," it admonishes, be "afraid to challenge and be assertive." Woe to the patient so weakened or distracted by his illness that he cannot follow such essential instructions or too confused to ask for the hospital fact sheet called "How to Avoid Medication Errors." Perhaps not making the most of such opportunities should now fall into the category of "noncompliance." But the expectation of this degree of cooperation couldn't have been predicted by Hippocrates himself, or even by the supernatural forethought ascribed to Aesculapius, the Greek god of medicine.

The awesome responsibilities that have recently dropped onto the weary shoulders of patients—and even onto the stalwart shoulders of those who try hard to remain well—have collectively been called "the tyranny of health." We are beset on all sides by rules we must follow lest dire consequences ensue. One form of such tyranny is manifested in the vaunted notion of autonomy, the darling of bioethicists and the source of so much conflict in the minds of physicians whose only motivation is to do the best they can for the men and women who look to them for help. There is such a thing as too much insistence on self-determination when health fails; it can indeed become a tyranny of unrealistic expectations for both the sick and the well. Though no one should doubt that the day of paternalistic medicine is long past, good sense should prevail if the very best and most humane of medical care is to be made available to every patient.

The essence of the Western medical tradition is, in the words of the ancient Hippocratic text *Precepts*, "love of mankind." Love of mankind, and of one another—by doctors, patients, and families—enables the mutual trust that leads to a partnership of shared responsibility and optimal decision making. This kind of love, it seems to me, prevents the tyranny not only of health but of paternalism and unbidden autonomy as well. And it does not put pressure or lay blame on the enervated sick, on the disadvantaged, or on those who, for whatever reason, are without the resources to "take charge" of their own health.

Of all the resounding nouns in the First Aphorism—"Life," "Art," "occasion," "experience," "judgment," "physician," "patient," "attendants," "externals"—the one whose applicability to the doctor is most controversial must surely be externals. In Hippocratic times, externals referred to the patient's surroundings: the general ambience most likely to encourage cure. A salubrious climate, good water, healthful and restorative food, an atmosphere of serenity—these were essential ingredients of the way of life that the Greeks called regimen. There was no disagreement about the physician's role in prescribing them. But in the late nineteenth century, medical reformers began to point out that disease is frequently the result of social conditions. This meant that doctors should not only become involved in matters of public health—such as water purification, safe housing, sewage disposal, immunizations, and the advocacy of personal cleanliness—but also work to advance social equality and relieve the conditions of the poor. Thus began a vigorous debate about the boundaries of medical responsibility, one that rages to the present day and will no doubt always rage. That society values the intervention of the profession in some of these matters is beyond doubt—one need only recall that the 1985 Nobel Peace Prize was awarded to an organization called International Physicians for the Prevention of Nuclear War.

But not all doctors, and certainly not all members of the general public, agree that white-coated influence is appropriate in such matters, and some argue strenuously against it. True, the followers of Hippocrates were committed to "make the externals cooperate," but of what should the externals consist today? What are their limits? How far should medicine—and, under its urging, society—go in imposing strictures on self-determination in the name of "taking charge of our own health"? It is one thing to legislate the listing of nutritional factors on food packages, another to impose a fiat banning junk-food machines from schools; it is one thing to demand that fast-food chains publish the caloric contents of their offerings, another to legislate the fat content of their hamburgers; it is one thing to print the surgeon general's warning on a pack of cigarettes, another to deprive someone of his right to light up in a public place; it is one thing to discourage smoking by taxing cigarettes out of proportion to their value, another to make the taxes so onerously high that many individuals are deprived of their free choice to indulge. In other words, it is one thing to oversee public and personal health in a free society, another to deprive people of the freedom to make their own decisions. As a physician committed to all the seemingly harsh dictates I have just listed, I nevertheless worry about the coercion that comes with such well-intended regulatory actions. It is a worry that has existed since the founding of our republic: how to balance the public welfare against the rights of the individual.

It is clear that the second sentence of the famed First Aphorism is far more problematic than the first. Whether the problem is the conundrum of autonomy or the question of how best to interpret the meaning of the word "cooperate," we physicians seem to waver in our conception of both authority and its limits. Here, as in so many other aspects of our calling, we practice the uncertain art.

Perhaps it is appropriate in this context to stop for a moment and consider the derivation of the word "physician," coming as it does from the Greek *physis*, meaning "nature": the essence of health was considered to be harmony with nature. But nature has another connotation. In preventing and treating illness, our constant companions and often our antagonists are human nature and the nature of personal liberty. As physicians, we ignore them to our peril, the peril of those we would help, and the peril of a free society.

THE ARTIST AND THE DOCTOR

The fine arts are timeless, but the Art is ever a creature of its time. In Latin, *ars* (singular) denotes a mental art involving knowledge or theory; *artes* (plural) denotes the fine arts. Since the earliest translation of classical texts into English, it has been customary to capitalize the word Art when the ancient authors referred specifically to the intellectual discipline we call medicine. Unlike the fine arts, the Art quickly becomes outdated and thereafter a matter of merely historical interest to only a few members of later generations.

Before Western doctors conversed in Latin, the languages in which their knowledge was conveyed were Arabic and Hebrew and, before that, Greek. It is to Greek that we must turn to find a word that applies to both the fine arts and the Art: *techne*, which means art that is useful, such as carpentry or shoemaking. The painter or sculptor requires techne to fulfill his vision; the physician has increasingly required techne—here read "technology"—to fulfill his mission.

As his use of technology increased, the physician considered himself less a practitioner of the Art and more an avatar of science. Today he likes to see himself as an applied scientist, safely distanced from the influences of subjectivity and emotion. But he labors under an illusion. His Art is no science. It is only by recognizing the truth of this predicament that he can attain the goal that originally attracted him to medicine: to be, first and foremost, a healer. The joy of medicine comes not only from relieving the suffering of one's fellows but from using one's judgment to deal with the uncertainties that hover over every bedside. In a sense, then, the practice of medicine is not only the Uncertain Art, but the Joyful Predicament. Therein lies its greatest challenge.

Almost since the period when Latin-speaking physicians were first spreading their Hippocratic doctrine throughout Europe, artists have been keeping a close watch on those who practice the Art. Sometimes in awe of the accomplishments of the physicians, sometimes exposing their pretensions, artists have left a record both of medicine's triumphs and of its follies. The catalogue of their names since the Renaissance is a long and distinguished one. Representing various eras are Albrecht Dürer, Hans Holbein the Younger, David Teniers, Rembrandt van Rijn, Joshua Reynolds, Francisco Goya, Luke Fildes, John Singer Sargent, Diego Rivera, Andrew Wyeth, and a host of caricaturists such as Thomas Rowlandson and Honoré Daumier. But no one has understood the mentality of the doctor as well as the nineteenth-century American artist Thomas Eakins. Specifically, it is his insight into the thicket of inconsistencies and vanity often called "the surgical personality" that brings his work to the level of genius. In his paintings, the Art is celebrated in all its distinction and exposed in all its presumptuousness.

The basis of my claim that Eakins is unrivaled in his perceptions of the contradictory strains in the character of so many doctors rests on two of his paintings. One is the magnificent work generally conceded to be his masterpiece, *The Portrait of Professor Gross*, or, as it later came to be called, *The Gross Clinic*. The other is *The Agnew Clinic*, another portrait of a leading American surgeon, painted fifteen years later, after Eakins had undergone vicissitudes in his career and personal life that may have made him a more sympathetic man.

Controversy over a new piece of art is hardly unknown. Three types of controversy seem to be the most prevalent: (1) the work introduces an entirely novel concept that flouts normative standards and is so alien to conventional thinkers that many refuse to accept it and some even deny that it is art at all; (2) the work is one in which the artist's deliberate intent is to shock, whether to make people think, to pull them out of complacency, or to deliver a message; (3) the work isn't created to produce a pother but it does, and its reception takes the artist by surprise. *The Gross Clinic* has traditionally been thought to fall into this final category, but that may be a misconception. Perhaps Eakins meant to shock; perhaps he was delivering a message not only to his viewers but to his subject as well.

The Gross Clinic had its origins in Philadelphia's 1876 United States Centennial Exposition, to all intents and purposes our nation's first world's fair. In conjunction with it, the American Medical Association hosted a meeting called the International Medical Congress. Seventy-one-year-old Dr. Samuel David Gross, professor of surgery at the city's Jefferson Medical College and president of the AMA, was unanimously elected president of the congress. Gross was indisputably the most prominent member of his specialty then practicing in the one-hundred-year-old nation—a claim he would surely have made for himself had not others made it for him. It is clear from reading his 855-page autobiography that he was not a modest man.

Gross was also proud of being the leading American opponent of the new concept of antisepsis, which had been promulgated in 1867 by Joseph Lister of the University of Edinburgh. Lister, perceptively interpreting Louis Pasteur's discovery that bacteria cause putrefaction in wine and beer, had shown that surgical infections were caused by similar microbes introduced into the wound at the time of operation. The combined contributions of these two inspired researchers led only a few years later to the germ theory of disease, destined to become the most transforming concept in medicine up to that time.

Samuel Gross did not believe in the power of germs. He denied that they played a significant role in infection, and he opposed Lister's advocacy of carbolic acid antisepsis as a means of destroying them. In this he was far from alone. For numerous reasons—not the least of which was inadequate grounding in science and microscopy—physicians in the United States and most of the countries of Europe, England included, refused to believe that invisible organisms were the cause of the massive postoperative infectious mortalities of those days. The death rate for Gross's institution is not known, but the figures cannot have been very different from those of the nearby Pennsylvania

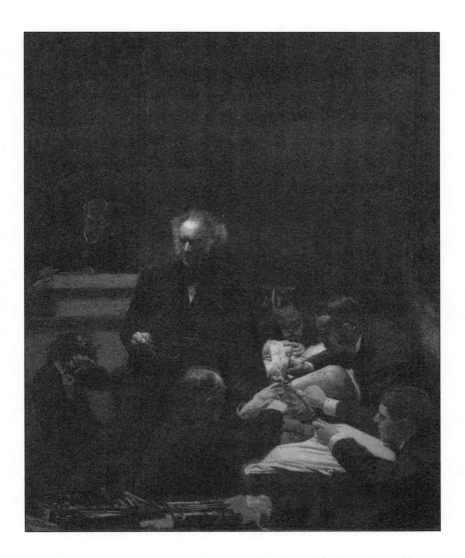

Thomas Eakins, *Portrait of Dr. Samuel D. Gross (The Gross Portrait).*

Hospital, where 27 percent of 152 amputees died between 1870 and 1874. These were typical statistics for American surgeons, but those from Europe were worse: they averaged more than 40 percent, almost all from infection.

So confident was Gross of his antigerm theory stance that he invited Lister to chair the congress's Section of Surgery, so that he might have a face-to-face opportunity to challenge the Englishman's views before a skeptical international audience whose French and German members would be the only ones prepared, by the superior development of science in their universities and hospitals, to embrace them. Lister delivered an eloquent three-hour oration but convinced none of his stubborn opponents, least of all the sublimely assured Gross. The precepts of the American mahatma continued to reign, and amputees continued to die in large numbers in Philadelphia and elsewhere, while Lister's mortality rates were consistently declining even lower than the 15 percent of the first series of antiseptic cases he had reported in 1867. It would be another decade before more progressive thinkers prevailed in American hospitals. By then, Samuel Gross was dead.

Thomas Eakins was certainly aware of this greatest of the controversies then roiling the international profession of medicine. His interest in the scientific study of the human body had been keen since his earliest days of training in 1864 and 1865, when, as a twenty-year-old student at the Pennsylvania Academy of the Fine Arts, he attended the anatomy classes of Dr. Joseph Pancoast, a professor of surgery at the Jefferson Medical College. Eakins's objective was to understand not only the structure of the human body but also its muscular functioning—a fascination he would avidly pursue for the rest of his career. He spent the years 1866 to 1869 in Paris, a city far more advanced in medical science than any save those in the German-speaking countries. Given his intellectual proclivities, he probably continued his scientifically based study of the body while he was there. He resumed his anatomical work in Philadelphia in the academic year 1873–74, the period during which he painted a portrait of Benjamin Howard Rand, professor of chemistry at the Jefferson Medical College. Eakins, known for developing a deep interest in the lives and accomplishments of his subjects, no doubt used the opportunity of being with Rand to further his scientific education. It is very likely that Rand discussed with him the interesting bacteriological work then being done by his fellow chemist Louis Pasteur. More important, though, the loud debate over Listerism, as the Englishman's doctrine was called, could be heard everywhere, especially in the precincts of the medical school so familiar to the artist. Eakins could not have avoided learning about the role of Samuel Gross in opposing it. It is inconceivable that the thirty-one-year-old painter had not formed an opinion of the theory's validity.

Eakins chose to portray Samuel Gross in the midst of an operation for osteomyelitis of the thigh, a crippling and often lethal infection of bone. While a bloody-handed assistant continues to probe the wound of the young patient, the noble-browed professor, knife held in his bare, crimson-soaked fingers, has paused portentously for a moment to turn to the assembled students in the surrounding gallery in order to declaim on some aspect of the operation. Though the students can be seen only in shadow, two figures are clearly visible in front of them. One is the artist himself, calmly sketching the scene from his seat in the first row of observers. The other is a woman clothed in a full-length black dress and bonnet, her work-worn hands held in a clawlike clench as though cringing from the horror she would have to witness were her averted face not covered by her tightly bent left arm. Very likely she is the patient's mother, unwillingly present to fulfill that era's notion of informed consent for charity patients.

There is not an iota of antisepsis in sight. Not only are the surgeon and his three assistants bare-handed, but over their shirts, waistcoats, and ties they are wearing ordinary frock coats, no doubt the same ones they don before every operation, rarely if ever cleaned of accumulated blood and pus. The unsterile surgical equipment lies on an exposed instrument case in the foreground, within easy reach of the unscrubbed hands that will use it. Lister be damned, the portrait seems to be proclaiming, and his germ theory with him.

The huge painting was startling, unlike anything that had been anticipated by those who had been waiting expectantly for Eakins to complete the great project he had undertaken. Aside from the many physicians who saw it as a tribute—to the eminence of Professor Samuel David Gross, to the ascendancy of Philadelphia medicine, and to the presumed growth of modern medical science in America—few observers failed to be shocked, specifically by the vivid images of blood, a terrified family member, and the patient's bare buttocks. *The Gross Clinic* was to be presented to the centennial exposition's selection committee for its celebratory American gallery of art, but when it was preliminarily displayed at the Haseltine Galleries in Philadelphia in 1875, the 96-by-78-inch painting aroused such a furor of outraged complaint that the committee decided it would be an inappropriate choice. The portrait, it was decreed, must hang elsewhere. Members of the International Medical Congress wishing to view it had to make their way to one of the surgical wards of the distant Army Post Hospital, located behind the city's U.S. Government Building.

Negative and even abusive criticism would follow the painting for many years. Decades later, when *The Gross Clinic* finally came to be accepted as the greatest of all depictions of our nation's medical scene, it was hailed as an encomium to a monumental figure in the history of American medicine, shown candidly in the fulfillment of his important work as a surgeon and teacher. Too graphic in 1876 for contemporary critics and a public unfamiliar with the hidden ways of operating theaters, the painting had nevertheless been immediately hailed by the alumni association of the Jefferson Medical College. In honor of their revered teacher, the group bought it from the artist for two hundred dollars in 1878 for presentation to their alma mater. For approximately a century, it hung in a place of distinction near the school's entrance hall, and it is now owned by the Philadelphia Museum of Art (at a cost of sixty-eight million dollars), though a replica hangs in the Eakins Gallery of the College's Jefferson's Alumni Hall. *The Gross Clinic* was the most popular feature of the much acclaimed Eakins exhibit mounted a few years ago at New York's Metropolitan Museum of Art. Though the painting won little honor in its time, its salience is now unquestioned.

* * *

What was it that Eakins really intended in his masterpiece? Was his purpose, in fact, to glorify Gross and the accomplishments of our nation's medicine at our centennial, as has universally been thought, or did he have an entirely different motive? Ponder something else: in depicting what observers have always considered to be his subject's grandeur and the profession's accomplishments and authority, Eakins was actually doing just the opposite. *The Gross Clinic* is in reality an exposé of the backwardness and smugly misguided self-aggrandizement in which American medicine was then wallowing, as exemplified by one of its most renowned professors. The fact that no one recognized it for what it was does not lessen the probability that the French-influenced, scientifically sophisticated painter deplored Gross's rejection of the germ theory and that the picture was his way of expressing it. In a word, I would suggest, *The Gross Clinic* was intended as a caricature. By capturing his subject's grandiose posture and superannuated methods, Eakins was portraying Gross as the pompous antediluvian he was later shown to be—the proprietor of a gross clinic indeed.

The absence of Eakins's name or any mention of the painting in the voluminous Gross autobiography may not be an oversight. Nor, I believe, is the absence of the words "antisepsis," "germ theory," and "carbolic acid" from the book's twelve-page index. Lister is mentioned only twice, each time in connection with one of the author's visits to Europe. A reader would never know that the brilliant Englishman had come to Philadelphia at Gross's invitation. I feel sure that America's leading surgeon came to realize, even if others did not, that he had been ridiculed by Eakins. I will go so far as to suggest that he may have recognized it immediately, and the banishment of the painting to a far-off venue was at the instigation of his powerful influence. At the very least (and evidence in his later writings supports this view), there can be little doubt that Gross had recognized the error of his anti-Listerism before his autobiography was published in 1887, by which time American acceptance of the germ theory had become the rule rather than the exception. It is of interest that the second volume of the autobiography uses *The Gross Clinic* as its frontispiece, which would seem to weaken my argument. Unfortunately for those who might think so, that second volume was published by his sons, from Gross's manuscript—three years after his death in 1884. He had no part in editing it or in decisions about its production, least of all in the choice of its frontispiece. In fact, it is well known that the man who inherited his surgical mantle at Jefferson, his son Samuel W. Gross, was convinced of Lister's theory and made good use of it. That theory would reach its ultimate victory with the opening of the aseptic operating rooms at the new Johns Hopkins Hospital in 1889, the same year in which Eakins painted his other great portrait of a famed American surgeon.

The Agnew Clinic presents a different picture entirely. Not only has the germ theory been accepted, but there is far less Moses-like glorification of the central figure. The seventy-one-year-old Hayes Agnew, professor of surgery at the University of Pennsylvania, has stepped back from the sterile operating scene and is wearily lecturing to a gallery of students in various stages of attention, including a few who are asleep. Unlike Gross, who at the same age was shown charged with the self-assured energy of a cynosure, Agnew looks like what he is: a tired old man near the end of his career. Once more, Thomas Eakins has looked deeply into a reality and laid bare the Art as only a master of *artes*—the fine arts—can do it. As Walt Whitman famously said of his friend and portraitist, "I never knew of but one artist, and that's Tom Eakins, who could resist the temptation to see what they think ought to be rather than what is. Eakins is not a painter, he is a force."

THE MAN OR THE MOMENT?

In a letter to the editor of *The New York Review of Books*, the eminent physicist and author Freeman Dyson was once taken to task for his essay on a new biography of Isaac Newton. "Dyson unfortunately shows how little versed he is in scholarship on Newton," wrote the correspondent, a faculty member of the Division of Humanities and Social Sciences at the California Institute of Technology. The basis for this denunciation was Dyson's apparent failure to realize that "historical research requires deep understanding of very different technical issues of long-gone science, together with substantial knowledge of social and cultural circumstances of the period." Though the writer went on to accuse Dyson of specific factual errors, he seemed most exercised by what he considered his quarry's misunderstanding of the era in which Newton had worked. The letter made me chuckle, and I'm certain that it had a similar effect on many other observers of the decades-long conflict between the social historians of science and those who might be termed the technical historians. In the unlikely event that the characteristically unflappable Dyson felt any heat from his antagonist's discontent, he might enjoy knowing that the temperature is even higher among scholars who study the history of medicine.

Until perhaps the 1960s, the technical historians of medicine dominated the field. They were almost all physicians, and hardly any of them had even the most minimal training in the formal methods of historical scholarship. Their interest was in the landmark achievements

This essay was chosen for inclusion in *The Best American Science and Nature Writing 2005*, edited by Jonathan Weiner (Houghton-Mifflin, 2005).

of clinical and laboratory medicine, and in the lives of the men—and very few women—responsible for them. To their self-appointed task they brought an expertise born of intensive medical training and extensive patient care. They focused only peripherally on wider historical currents. These doctors were, in the strictest sense of the word, amateurs. When they slipped away from their consulting rooms to dusty library stacks—or when they elected to forgo Caribbean vacations in favor of research trips to old hospitals in far-off countries— they did it for love of the grand tradition of their forebears, to which they considered themselves heir.

Things began to change in the 1950s, as the field of medical history became increasingly professionalized. After that time, the academic degree held by authors of scholarly articles was as likely to be Ph.D. as MD, and before long the former predominated. Within twenty years, the majority of participants in the annual meeting of the American Association for the History of Medicine had earned doctorates in history. Among the most prominent were men and women who held both titles and had abandoned patient care to devote most or all of their time to historical studies.

With this shift came a change in focus from the technical and personal to the societal and cultural. No longer was it sufficient to investigate the exploration and the explorer; the intellectual atmosphere of an entire era was now scrutinized. Medical science was seen as the product less of individual genius than of the Zeitgeist. Discoverers were shaped by their times, not the reverse.

The bedside doctors welcomed these new insights, but they were not happy to watch their perspectives being shoved aside by people with little or no clinical background. Though both medical doctors and social historians have something valid to say, the latter are currently in the ascendancy. The old-style physician-historians have been routed, and in the process, much has been lost.

By 1980, Leonard Wilson of the University of Minnesota, a Ph.D. and the editor of the *Journal of the History of Medicine and Allied Sciences*, warned of the consequences of a history grounded completely in cultural causes and dominated by scholars who "see little of the laboratory and less of the clinic." He said of such scholars, "They tend to neglect questions of clinical medicine, of the biology of disease, and of science, even when such questions had a direct bearing on the particular historical subject with which they are concerned. The result is incomplete and sometimes severely distorted history. . . . If such social history be considered medical history, . . . it is medical history without medicine."

And one might add that it is medical history without the colorful characters who made it. Beyond a doubt, there exists a cultural inevitability to scientific discovery. The sun would have been recognized as the center of our solar system whether or not Copernicus had lived, and probably soon after he published his monumental *De revolutionibus orbium coelestium* in 1543; the debunking of the phlogiston theory was in the cards, and Lavoisier merely speeded the process; the discovery of the structure of DNA would have taken only a few more months had not Watson and Crick outsprinted everyone else to the finish line. In each case, the times were ready; the ambient culture and the state of contemporary science virtually ensured that these advances would occur, and fairly soon.

At least in medicine, the precedents were in place for every discovery by the time it was presented. Even the transcendent contributions of Harvey and Pasteur would have been made had those two brilliant men never been born, though they would have taken place somewhat later. But they would have been made in a different way, usually as the result of a different process—because part of the process is the distinctive personality of the discoverer.

Far more often than most social historians are willing to admit, a discovery made at a particular time and place—and the form in which it is brought to the community of medical thinkers—is unique to the person who is responsible for it. Not only that, but it not uncommonly arises from the idiosyncrasies of that one individual and may even be the expression of his or her personality, background, or personal situation. Similarly, when a contribution is not readily accepted, the failure can often be ascribed as much to the way the innovator has come to it and brought it to attention as to a cultural milieu not yet ready to embrace it. Of all that is "incomplete" and "severely distorted," and of all that is lost by the social historian's downplaying of individual effort in favor of surrounding influences, the one missing factor that most diminishes the ultimate narrative is the unique personality of the contributor and the ways in which it plays into the process of discovery and the overall cavalcade of history.

Regardless of the surrounding culture, some scientists are aggressive while others are mild-mannered; some are resentful of authority while others do precisely what their teachers expect; some are intolerant of delay while others achieve their ends through patient persistence. These characteristics profoundly affect the nature and timing of landmarks in medicine. When Thomas Carlyle wrote that "history is the essence of innumerable biographies," he was referring specifically to the role of inimitable individuality in shaping the events of our world. Even today, when discoveries are often team efforts, it is ultimately the single observer or experimenter who must initiate the process of his or her own contribution to science. The fact that the same contribution would eventually have been made by someone else does not in the least vitiate the force of that truth.

Examples abound. Throughout the twenty-five-hundred-year history of Western scientific medicine, progress has repeatedly been spurred or slowed by the personal behavior of an individual. Most prominent in this regard during the classical period was Galen of Pergamon, the second-century physician whose many public demonstrations of animal experimentation energized the doctors of his time and explained physiological phenomena previously obscured by a hodgepodge of spurious theories. So powerful was the effect of his research, his public performances, and the many dozens of books he left to posterity that his influence towered over the meager efforts of his successors. But Galen was a vain, fiercely competitive self-promoter, driven as much by the search for eternal glory as by the search for knowledge. Summoning all the authority he had earned from his scientific and clinical contributions, he declared that his teachings were to be regarded as the unchanging gospel of medicine. There was no point, he taught his eager acolytes, in attempting to seek new information about health, disease, or the structure and function of the human body; he had created a complete and sufficient system of medicine.

Such was the forcefulness of Galen's personality, as expressed both during his life and through the enduring influence of his writings, that his teachings were blindly followed for nearly a millennium and a half. Medicine stagnated in his honor until the sixteenth century. At that point, along came Andreas Vesalius, an ambitious and endlessly curious young man as contentious as his Greek predecessor. Among Vesalius's most striking personality characteristics was a love-hate attitude toward authority figures that culminated again and again in angry conflict. He stood up to his teachers, first at the University of Paris, then at Bologna and Padua. Finally, he took on Galen himself, denouncing the ancient master for the more than two hundred errors he had made in his anatomical descriptions and exposing the reason: all of Galen's work had been done on monkeys and dogs. In 1543, at the age of twenty-eight, Vesalius published his monumental book *De humani corporis fabrica*, which founded the scientific study of anatomy and established for medicine the principle that progress can be made only by taking tiny steps—and by challenging authority. Henceforth, medical innovators would abandon the old reliance on the conception of grand theories into which observations must be uncomfortably pigeonholed.

In my own specialty, surgery, there are abundant examples of men whose personalities left their mark on the course of medical history, Zeitgeist or no Zeitgeist. In 1837, a young Hungarian obstetrician named Ignác Semmelweis, in a moment of inspired brilliance, discovered the reason why almost 20 percent of the obstetric patients in virtually all of the major European hospitals were dying of childbed fever: the obstetricians were not washing their hands after performing autopsies on the pus-ridden bodies of the women who had died of the same disease within the previous twenty-four hours. Without a microscope and long before germs were recognized as the agents of disease, Semmelweis intuited that "invisible organic matter" on the hands of the doctors was being conveyed into the genital tracts of women in labor, consigning them to an anguished death. But he was a self-righteous and combative man, and he alienated his superiors and most of his colleagues by accusing them, when they would not accept his theory without experimental proof, of remorselessly murdering women. After a halfhearted attempt to provide such evidence using a few rabbits, he refused to do further laboratory work, contemptuously declaring the truth of his assertion to be so self-evident that no additional studies were needed. He saw every attack on his doctrine as an attack on himself. Semmelweis would die in a Vienna mental asylum, most probably beaten to death by orderlies trying to restrain him. His great discovery was forgotten, and the promulgation of the germ theory, which could have occurred around 1840 had he been less bullheaded, was delayed until 1867.

When the theory was finally brought forth in that year by the gentle, supremely patient Quaker surgeon Joseph Lister, the notion of microscopic organisms causing disease seemed so outlandish—and even foolish—to the physicians of the time that it found little general acceptance. It was the quiet persistence and good-natured equanimity of Lister—along with his continuing experiments, his demonstrations, his writings, and his willingness to travel from hospital to hospital and from country to country, to disseminate his beliefs—that finally won the day, though that day was delayed for some two decades.

Two more examples from widely separated historical periods illustrate the significance of the role sometimes played by an innovator's personality, each presented independently of the era and aura in which he worked. The first is the story of an introverted, asthenic little Breton physician, René-Théophile-Hyacinthe Laënnec, who stood five feet three inches tall and, at the age of thirty-five, had never spent an hour alone in the company of a woman who was not a relative or a servant. One day in 1816, on hospital rounds, Laënnec faced the terrifying obligation of putting his ear—in the manner of the time—directly against the chest of an intimidatingly pretty young woman in order to hear the transmitted sounds of her lung and heart disease. The pathologically shy little man backed off and hurried home. En route, he chanced upon some boys playing a game familiar to him, in which the scratchings of a pin on one end of a long rod of wood were interpreted by a lad listening at the other. Struck with inspiration, he hurried back to the hospital, rolled up a sheaf of papers into a cylinder, placed it under the left breast of the amused girl—and in that historic moment invented the instrument he called *le baton,* soon to be refined into what we now know as the stethoscope. Laënnec carved his own *batons,* which could be purchased for three francs as a sort of supplement to the thirteen-franc book he would write three years later, describing the many uses of his new diagnostic tool.

The second example is culled from the annals of American medicine. William Halsted, a brilliant and dashing young New York surgeon known for his speed and technical derring-do in the operating room—as well as for his high living—was among the first experimenters with cocaine after it was shown, in 1884, to induce local anesthesia when injected into skin or muscle. Having no idea of the drug's dangers, Halsted used himself as an experimental subject and soon became our nation's inaugural cocaine addict. Following a long period of attempted recovery, he secured an appointment as the first professor of surgery at the new Johns Hopkins Medical School shortly after it opened in Baltimore in 1893. Halsted emerged from the darkness of his cocaine-saturated period as a very different man from the fearless risk taker of his early career: a methodically slow, meticulous operator whose painstaking methods would be emulated by the many surgeons he trained. The so-called Halstedian technique in time spread throughout the country and made possible a new "surgery of safety," as it became known, and the introduction of many innovative operations that required great gentleness and minute attention to detail. This withdrawn, asocial professor is remembered today as the father of American surgery. His methods of dealing with tissues and organs, essential if further progress was to be made, would not have been introduced for years or even decades had it not been for the personality alteration that resulted from their inventor's cocaine addiction.

Though my own fascination with medical history lies mostly with the people who have made it, I would never claim that this perspective is always the most effective one. Several factors—social, cultural, technological, and personal—can be explored separately, and for the sake of analysis they may be treated as independent variables. Nevertheless, the process of discovery arises from all of them working together, each in its proper proportion. Some variables may be more consequential than others in any given case, but they are all crucial to the evolution of the bit of progress being studied. The punishment for devaluing the significance of any of them is the writing of bad history.

LETTERS FROM A
HEART TRANSPLANT CANDIDATE

For me to live, someone has to die. That's a very complex thought. It deals in a way with a form of ethics. Is it right to want to live at the expense of others' grief, to pray that I am found a strong young heart when I know full well that it was part of a body that was younger, stronger and had more years to give than I will ever have? It's not difficult to rationalize these thoughts away with statistics, to take a position that it's better I should live than no one. But these thoughts are real and they have to be faced and not superficially. Science had made me a potential recipient of a modern miracle. In a sense it's a blessing and one which I will always treat accordingly. To do less is beyond my conception.

The author of these words was fifty-six years old when he wrote them in January 1988. He had been waiting for a heart transplant since the previous September.

I had known George Leyden only a month at that time. Our relationship had begun as a kind of blind date, arranged by his cardiologist at the Yale–New Haven Hospital. In background, personality, interests, life experiences—even body build—the two of us could not have been more at opposite poles had we been bred for the characteristics that made us so different from each other. What we shared was a worldview. But it will always remain a mystery to me how two men born only a few months apart could have come to precisely the same place in significant areas of their personal philosophies when they had traveled such dissimilar paths to get there—and started their journeys at such different points and under such different circumstances. But perhaps I am only flattering myself. There was a deep vein in George's keen perception of himself and the events swirling around him—events over which he had little control but that would nevertheless determine his fate—that was his alone. Few of us dare presume to claim such understanding.

It hardly mattered that our journeys had been so dissimilar. I was fascinated by George, and for some unfathomable reason he seems to have been equally fascinated by me. Opposites are said to attract. For George Leyden and me, the mutual magnet lay at some midpoint between our vastly separated experiences of life and drew us together with a force not only powerful but against which neither of us had any intention of resisting. But great as was the energy of our attraction, death would prove to be stronger. George never got his transplant. He died almost eight months after writing me that letter in which he wrestled with his feelings of ambivalence and guilt.

But during that brief period of time, George revealed himself to me in ways that some of my oldest friends have never been able to do, or I to them. Perhaps because courage came so easily to him, he was unafraid to be afraid; perhaps because good luck had accompanied him all his life, he was aware that it might desert him when he most needed it; perhaps because success had been his almost for the asking, he was willing to acknowledge, albeit only at rare moments, that this time he might fail; perhaps because optimism and self-confidence were so natural a part of his makeup, he was willing to speak about morbid thoughts and inner conflicts. In agreeing to my request that he write the series of contemplations that he would entitle "The Musings of a Heart Transplant Candidate"—which in time would amount to more than eighty closely typed pages documenting his thoughts on every day from our meeting until the week before he died—he entered a pact with me, and kept his part of the bargain with a grace and honesty that fulfilled criteria reminiscent of those described by Jean Jacques Rousseau in his own *Confessions*: "I have entered on an enterprise which is without precedent, and will have no imitator. I propose to show my fellows a man as nature made him, and this man shall be myself."

I don't know that the "Musings" had no precedent, and they certainly have had plenty of unknowing imitators. But what really counts here is the man. Hamlet's "I shall not look upon his like again" might have been said of anyone, for each of us is unique. But we know what Shakespeare meant by those words, and that is precisely what I mean, too, when I say the same of my friend.

The blind date that brought us together in mid-December 1987 was the result of a shared pragmatism. I was planning to write an article for *The New Yorker* that would explain cardiac transplantation to a general reader; George was an active participant in the campaign to publicize the problems inherent in obtaining sufficient donor organs. Each of us fit well into the other's packet of needs. We met at the suggestion of Dr. Lawrence Cohen, the chief of cardiology at Yale.

The organ procurement team at Yale–New Haven Hospital had been eager to enroll George in their efforts to publicize the need for donors. He was a senior executive at IBM, an articulate, accomplished communicator, and a man of keen intelligence, whose well-honed ability to explicate complex matters in clear language was characterized by a notable absence of talking down to his listeners. It didn't hurt that he was six feet two inches tall, handsome in a classically distinguished and yet remarkably youthful way, and in every sense fulfilled the image of the former college varsity athlete and naval aviator that he was. When Larry Cohen told me about him, I was sure that such a man was too good to be true.

Beyond being an enthusiastic spokesman for the cause of organ donation, George was planning an innovative project to be carried out after he had received his transplant: he would launch a program in which major corporations would enroll potential donors among their employees, in the same way they had long been conducting company blood drives.

George's cardiac problems seem to have begun about ten years prior to his being placed on the transplant list, when he returned exhausted from a three-week business trip to the Far East and Latin America. He slept badly his first night home, awoke early the next morning, and went jogging in the streets of his Stamford, Connecticut, neighborhood. To his surprise, he found himself having difficulty breathing and soon became aware of an irregular heartbeat. Over the following three months, his episodes of shortness of breath became more frequent, and he finally called for an appointment to see his family physician. The diagnosis made on that very first visit was cardiomyopathy, a generic term for any progressive process that gradually impairs the functioning of the muscular walls of the ventricles, the two powerful pumping chambers of the heart.

The various causes of cardiomyopathy are spread across a wide spectrum, ranging from coronary artery obstruction to viruses, drugs such as alcohol and cocaine, and a variety of underlying diseases. The basis of George's problem was never discovered. Although he admitted that the intense demands of his job had led to too much drinking and smoking, a viral explanation seemed most likely. For several years, he had been directing a program designed to enhance the skills of IBM employees in Canada, Latin America, and the Far East, a total of forty-five countries. The work had been exciting, the atmosphere heady, and the stress extraordinary as he traveled again and again through seventeen time zones, visiting nations inhabited by two-thirds of the earth's population. Not only did he find himself susceptible to the temptations of alcohol and tobacco on those long missions far from home, but the hectic pace of his life meant that he was at added risk for the predations of ever-present viral agents as well.

The day George went to his doctor was also the first day of his life that he had ever missed from work. Shortly afterward, on September 21, 1977, he was seen in consultation at the Yale–New Haven Hospital by Dr. Cohen, who would thereafter be his cardiologist. Placed on a program of rest and medications to strengthen his heartbeat, regulate its rhythm, and prevent fluid retention, he spent three months gradually recovering until he was finally able to return to IBM, the company he had joined as a telephone switchboard dispatcher upon leaving the Navy in the mid-1950s. Because his activities were now permanently restricted, the rapid upward course of his career had ended. IBM did everything it could to find a suitable job for him within the organization, but to no avail. It was finally decided that he would take a paid two-year leave of absence under an Executive Loan Program, to become a consultant to the president of Sarah Lawrence College. As George would later put it, "I learned a lot, they learned a lot, and I left with friends who will remain with me forever."

When the two years were over, several assignments for IBM followed, involving consultation work in educational programs and then a position in which George briefed executives for some of the company's major accounts. Finally, he was handed the responsibility for supervising the design, construction, and implementation of a new $150 million facility in Thornwood, New York, that would consolidate all of the company's domestic customer executive education.

Until shortly before I met George, in December 1987, he had been at that job for three years. But the long period of progressive cardiomyopathy had taken its toll. His heart was enlarging as its muscle gradually deteriorated. Finally, the worsening disability had forced him to turn over the leadership of the project to a colleague, relegating himself to a consultant's position in which he came to work only one day a week.

By that time, George's cardiac function was weakening rapidly. Between February and August 1987, there had been a marked increase in his heart's size and a worsening of symptoms. In mid-September, he was admitted for a week to the Yale–New Haven Hospital, where studies showed a significant decline in the percentage of blood that his failing left ventricle was able to pump out. With the situation on such a marked downhill course in spite of the finest medical care and the patient's strict adherence to the management plan, there was no choice but to recommend that a cardiac transplant be done. After the entire clearance process of social, financial, and psychological considerations had been completed, George's name was put on the list and the long wait began.

The succinctness of the social worker's note managed by its professional flatness to obscure the dramatic reality of that instant in George's journey: "Mr. Leyden appears to be an excellent candidate for heart transplant. He is highly motivated, has a good support system and strong goals for a satisfying future with his family." A man's life was being described in those two emotionless sentences, and the patterns of the road he had traversed to reach that day.

For one thing, the support system was more than merely strong.

Not only was it watertight, but it had been securely in place for more than three decades and growing steadily more sturdy. In 1955, the Navy had transferred George to the Canal Zone from a posting in Trinidad, where he was serving as a pilot in one of the last of the old seaplane squadrons. Shortly after arriving, "I fell in love with the most beautiful girl I had ever seen," a young woman living near the base with her government-employed parents. The competition for her attention was keen, but George was undaunted. "I began to plan my marriage strategy, in spite of all the odds against it." Though "[e]very single male in the area whose hormones were flowing in the right direction had eyes for Helen," our hero, as was his lifelong custom, prevailed. The couple were married in May 1956. The radiance of that day can only be imagined as a novelist might have written about it—the dashing young naval officer resplendent in full uniform, taking as his bride "the most beautiful girl I had ever seen."

Shortly afterward, Lieutenant Commander Leyden began jet training in Pensacola, Florida, where his plans for a naval career were to receive a shocking jolt. As he casually watched from the porch of the Officers Club one sunny Sunday morning while enjoying a leisurely brunch, a close friend took off in a plane whose engine he was testing, with all of its crew aboard. Without warning or apparent reason, the plane suddenly lost power and crashed into a breakwater that the pilot was desperately attempting to clear. "In the space of less than a minute, this idyllic picture was transformed into a thunderous cauldron of fire, destruction and death. . . . All but one of the crew was instantly killed and my feelings about flying, the Navy and my future took a one hundred and eighty degree turn." He left the service, took an entry-level job with IBM, and began his rapid ascent through the ranks.

The result of George's happy marriage would be a happy home with four happy children. "Our house was always filled with other people's kids; there was usually a lot of laughter, a lot of fun and a lot going on all the time." When I later met the Leydens, three of their children were married and the fourth was engaged. All of them were living within easy driving distance of one another, so that the closeness of a single large extended family remained intact. There were six grandchildren.

Such was the state of grace of George Leyden in November 1987, when our lives began their brief period of being intertwined: in religion a committed Catholic, in politics a staunch Republican, in life a fulfilled human being—but for his cardiomyopathy. He was a successful man with a failed heart.

When I met George, he was exactly as Larry Cohen had described him. Except for a cautious deliberateness in locomotion to avoid shortness of breath, there was nothing about him to suggest that the structure ticking so inefficiently in his chest was as much a time bomb as a faltering heart. Our first meeting was over coffee in the hospital cafeteria. To anyone who may have seen us that day, we must have appeared to be two conservatively dressed middle-aged physicians in serious and deep discussion about the management of some patient's clinical problem. Or perhaps not so serious and not so deep, because from time to time we interrupted ourselves by amused smiles and even a few soft bursts of laughter. Even at that first encounter, we were enjoying the touch of wryness that found its way into each other's sense of humor.

George's manner had none of the guardedly formal tone I would have associated with the personality of a senior executive in a Fortune 500 corporation. Quite the opposite—he was disarmingly open, and as genuinely curious about me as I was about him. Though he was the putative center of interest as a transplant candidate, I had the feeling that at the end of our journey together *he* might just as well have been planning to make *me* the topic of a published article about surgeons. Had I known the luminous quality of the writing I would soon be receiving from him, I might have, in fact, suggested that we turn the tables on each other.

I made two requests of George. The first was that he write a biographical sketch to bring me up to the present, so that I might better understand the background not only of his illness but of his attitudes and responses to the events that would be taking place over the following months. The second was that he periodically sit down at his computer (IBM had provided him with what was then its most advanced model, so that he could work at home with a maximum of effortless efficiency) and simply allow himself to free associate—let his mind wander over the events he was experiencing and record them as though he were telling them to me in ordinary conversation. And of course, we would meet from time to time and also speak on the phone.

This was precisely the physical form our relationship would take. George sent me the first of the series of letters shortly after New Year's of 1988, dated "at random from 12/21/87 to 1/2/88." It consisted of eighteen pages of single-spaced narrative, describing the colorful life of a colorful man. From then onward, the missives would come periodically, always having been written over the course of a few days to a week or so, detailing the events of that period and George's thoughts about them. As the theme for the first of what he called "The Musings of a Heart Transplant Candidate," George chose a stanza from Longfellow:

> Let us, then be up and doing,
> With a heart for any fate;
> Still achieving, still pursuing,
> Learn to labor and to wait.

To "wait." Ironically, the word shares its Indo-European origin with "vigor" and "liveliness," of which George had long been deprived. But "vigil," too, comes from the same root, and vigil is what I now began to share with George, although only in the most peripheral sense. For who can really share the awe-filled loneliness of a man awaiting a young and healthy heart with the knowledge that his own poor cardiac mechanism may not be able to sustain him until it can be found? Perhaps there are some who can, at least to an extent: most of all those who have loved him, and perhaps also a new friend, whose feelings of concern and loyalty nevertheless cannot but remain intermixed with a writer's self-interest—a fact of which both George and I were acutely aware although it was never spoken between us. A thing that *was* spoken between us was the statistic that hovered over the vigil like a dark and lowering cloud: in 1987, at least a third of American transplant-eligible patients with end-stage disease were dying before a suitable donor heart could be found. (Most recently, in early 2007, the figure is closer to 50 percent. Though cardiac care has improved, the availability of donor hearts has decreased by approximately 20 percent.) As George had told a reporter interviewing him for *The New York Times*, "Sooner or later . . . the race becomes very dramatic. Will you find a heart before the patient dies? The last thing I want is for that not to happen." Yet it did.

It strikes me as I prepare these pages, which are meant as both a narrative and a tribute to my friend, that he speaks for himself far better than my inadequate words and an occasional quote can convey. What follows, therefore, is a series of excerpts from his letters to me and also brief sections of his "Musings." As must have been said to him many times while he was flying airplanes for the Navy, "Over to you, Leyden."

As George waited, he pondered over waiting:

> I know of few people who excel at waiting (a religious fanatic perhaps, a martial arts devotee, a duck hunter) and I imagine most share my impatience to some degree. Incidentally, I define patience as a form of despair that we often disguise as a virtue. [January 8–12]

A few weeks later, he wrote of the responses his illness was eliciting in some of the staff and his colleagues at IBM:

> Because I am now "different" from virtually all other people that most have as friends or acquaintances, I'm treated accordingly by everyone. There are elements of fear, lack of knowledge and sympathy all interacting and it results initially in a strained, but very gentle atmosphere. I've become fragile in everyone's eyes and a person, while not to be pitied, to be treated somehow differently than before. No one really knows what to do. . . . [E]veryone I deal with goes out of their way to be nice, to be pleasant, to be warm and concerned. . . . No one chooses to argue for fear of injuring my psyche and possibly doing damage to my poor dilapidated heart. In meetings, people are

careful that my chair is well placed and comfortable. Coffee or re-freshments are at my instant beck and call. My counsel is earnestly solicited and listened to. [People] are thoughtful and kind and cour-teous and obedient. Isn't it unfortunate one has to be ill to cause such a generous response?

The minuses are patently obvious. I, by necessity, question the sincerity of even close friends. I don't mean to imply that my associ-ates are being pleasant to the detriment of how they really feel, but I firmly believe that the current lack of healthy disagreement could well produce a less viable end result. In the meantime, however, going to the office in my current condition is kind of fun! [Janu-ary 13–16]

And a few days later:

Recently, however, things have been getting a little difficult. The "waiting" is taking its toll. My fuse is a little shorter, my patience is wearing thin and my anxiety is becoming visible. The most frequent comments from work associates have to do with "how well I'm bear-ing up under what must be such a terrific strain" and I'm getting a little tired of hearing it. They mean well and it's not an unfair obser-vation. I've always had the ability to hide anguish. If a situation really hurts, I can block it out. I don't cry at funerals; I rarely cry at all except in front of my wife (not my children, just my wife). My other emotions are less well controlled—anger, joy, pleasure—but because I rarely show fear or sadness, I've garnered a reputation for strength. My friends, associates, even my family think of me as a "rock," the guy who never gets "shook up." In a sense it's a sincere compliment. It's also a burden. . . .

Death is not an overriding concern. It has some personal overtones I don't relish, but I can push those aside. It's the weakening of my spirit that bothers me. I simply can't allow myself to be anything but a role model patient. Actually, I don't know how else to act. I despise weakness in others. To allow myself even a moment of doubt or self pity would be unconscionable, so I don't. My wonderful wife says that I won't allow anything bad to happen to me. She really believes that. I hope I warrant that faith. . . . [January 13–16]

And then a week later:

I have very little experience waiting for things and while I frequently advise my family and business associates to "have patience," that everything will work out for the best, I'm a poor practitioner. For years I've been on the offensive, gathering a reputation as a doer, a person who makes things happen. . . . I now find myself practicing that particular thing that I despise the most—*waiting for something to happen.* My temper flares when I have to wait for even minutes. To wait for days or weeks (now months) is something with which I am not familiar. I despise it. I'm trying to do it with style (smiling, joking, acting as though my days are nothing unusual) and to some extent, I'm succeeding. It's a facade, a practiced piece of behavior that looks normal to all but my family and closest friends who can quickly spot the chinks. But I'm tired of it and as of now, I'm changing my approach to the problem. [January 17–24]

George's change consisted of determining in his own mind that the transplant would take place during the first two weeks of February. Accustomed to making sweeping plans and then overseeing every detail until final completion, he used this formulation as his magical way of assuring that he would get a heart—and soon. But like the military man and corporate executive he was, he had a contingency plan in mind should things not happen according to his projection:

And if for some reason a proper donor isn't available before Saint Valentine's Day, I will restructure my plans for yet another date. But I'll be damned if I'm going to continue this daily/nightly anxiety ritual any more. It's simply too exhausting. [January 17–24]

The inaction of a man who had spent his life at the forefront of action, and the dragging of the seemingly endless days one after another, stimulated half-awake nocturnal imaginings of high drama:

I'm having trouble getting to sleep or returning to sleep if I wake during the night. I fantasize when I should be dozing off. There's no consistency to my fantasies save the fact that they are always action oriented. I run, jump, save damsels in distress, rescue hostages; always high adventure of a sort and in great detail. To stop it, I turn on the light and read. . . . [W]hen (that's the word—WHEN—) I'm blessed with a new heart, my fantasies will recede and I then, in fact, may be able to rescue a few damsels, assuming they don't run too fast and really want to be rescued. [January 17–24]

Any opportunity for activity was an opportunity eagerly embraced, to change the fallow pattern of disengagement and disperse the empty sense of uselessness. The one day of work was the high point of the week. The moment he got into his car on each of those much anticipated mornings, George could feel himself change:

Suddenly I'm comfortable. I'm going somewhere, I'm preparing to do something constructive. When I arrive at my destination, my energy level is high, my interest is piqued and I thoroughly enjoy whatever is facing me. I'm no longer sick. I'm a vital, contributing individual and feel wonderful. . . . I feel I can do more than I'm doing, but then I'm reminded that my left ventricular ejection fraction is twelve percent. . . . [Though called a "fraction," this assessment of cardiac performance is, in fact, expressed as a decimal and is equivalent to the percentage of the blood in its fully filled chamber that the ventricle is capable of pumping forth with each contraction. The normal figure averages 65 percent. A recent textbook of medicine states, "(I)n severe heart failure, the ejection fraction may be reduced to less than 0.20," which gives some idea of how badly George's heart was performing.] It infuriates me. . . . I don't like being ill. I've never been ill. Coping with it is a challenge I fear I'm failing. My impatience is methodically driving me wild. I wonder if I'm learning something from all of this? I certainly hope so. If mental agony can create a better man, it won't be long before I'm one terrific guy. [January 17–24]

Aggravating the long days was the frustration engendered by the scarcity of donor hearts, because the mechanisms for obtaining them were faulty:

I understand that under the best of circumstances, no more than fifteen to eighteen hundred transplants will take place during 1988. [At present, more than 2,200 hearts are being transplanted each year in the United States.] I also hear that the demand will exceed the supply by a factor of five or six. . . . This situation is wrong. Hundreds, probably thousands of people die in hospitals, of all places, that are unsolicited donor candidates. Other hundreds of people die annually (needlessly, but it happens) on the nation's highways. Most, by far, are unsolicited donor candidates. . . . We wait until [people] die, and then ask. Now that makes a hell of a lot of sense, doesn't it? The donor is deceased; what in God's name does he or she care? So we ask their next of kin, their traumatized loved ones, if they would consent to the cannibalizing of their lost companion. The mere fact that we've got the gall to ask is a bit sick in itself. That the answer is usually "no" is completely understandable, logical and ridiculously predictable.

What's the AMA doing about this? What government programs exist? Is private industry involved in any way? [A] lot of years in our enlightened society tell me that I'm going to be dissatisfied with the answers I get. Today I'm in no position to make my presence felt in this arena. Tomorrow, and I pray tomorrow comes quickly, you are going to hear from me. I can't do it alone—but I can raise a lot of ruckus! [January 25–31]

From time to time, George would remark on some of the touching things that were said to him by friends and colleagues, and the awkward comments, too. Like so many of the brave whose courage is so seamlessly interwoven into their characters, he was surprised when it was mentioned:

I was called "courageous" a few weeks ago by an individual who knows my situation but not my personality. . . . That's a misnomer.

I'm protective, honest and reasonably moral. I would kill or die for my family and given good cause, for my country. This has little to do with bravery. In my thinking, it has to do with being idealistic, a bit starry-eyed and maybe old-fashioned. Too bad these virtues seem strange to many of our politicians. . . . We certainly lack for role models in Washington.

I remain stable and "well compensated" (a wonderfully ambiguous medical term that means absolutely nothing to me) according to the good Dr. Cohen. I suspect I'm not getting appreciably worse or someone would tell me. I do know I'm being stretched out far further than anyone should. It's not pleasant for me and it's an unadulterated hardship on my family. . . . I know [that each one of my associates] feels sorry for me and that in itself is a terrible situation. It's difficult, my friend, and while I'm a fairly strong character blessed with a good sense of humor, I'd rather be tested in other ways. Let me know if you would like to get together. I don't know what we'd talk about; you know more about me than anyone save my spouse, but I need a change of scenery. What I really need is a strong young heart preferably from a larger black woman. Can you imagine the fun I could have in that situation? It would drive the staid corporation personnel department absolutely wild. [March 2–23]

As the months dragged on, contingency plans were forgotten and there was only the waiting.

For the past two nights, I have been awakened by a telephone ring in my dreams. I then anxiously wait for my wife to officially wake me to get ready for our Yale–New Haven trip. Nothing happens. To wait endlessly for something that seems never to occur is a draining experience. No one save my enemies should have to do this. And I can't even think of an enemy I would wish it on. [February 17–25]

From time to time, George would comment on how time had elided into endless time. He began his April 3 letter with

My God, it's springtime. This dratted affliction of mine has taken a perfectly good fall and winter out of my life and left few fond memories. The good things were having the time to take stock of myself, meeting some (not many) memorable new people, . . . gaining a measure of relief from the burdens of daily business pressures (a mixed reward) and confirming that those half dozen or so souls I count as true friends, really are. [March 24–April 2]

As time passed, it was becoming increasingly difficult to keep up the appearance of being a man whose equanimity was sufficient to carry him through situations in which the average person would succumb to the inner turmoil and drown in it. A springtime cold worsened the usual shortness of breath, and George wondered how long he could continue to struggle with his desperate need to remain in control of himself:

I cannot allow myself to weaken in appearance or attitude (spirit) in front of my peers or family for fear that something terrible will happen. The fact that nothing of significance will happen whether I come or go is something I have great difficulty with. This is precisely the situation I wanted to create and now, having done so, I can't seem to live with it. The drain is having to appear certain and confident about everything I do when in reality I sometimes have real fears and am not certain or confident about anything.

And that's why I'm feeling out of sorts right now. . . . Usually my family and friends know the reasons when I'm upset. At the moment their reactions to those reasons are flavored with honest sorrow and concern and while those are kind and loving thoughts, I despise them. If someone would abrasively tell me to sit down and shut up, my response would probably be to do so; but no one ever tells me to. . . .

Friday, I spent an hour or two with Larry Cohen. I cherish these visits even if, as now, he has little encouraging news. His inquiry as to my general well-being was met with a response he has seldom heard from me. All the bravado that I spill out to the general public (and to some extent, my own family) dissolved, as it should. . . . Am I alarmed—you bet your bippy! With the kind of logic that emanates from fear, I decide I've either taken a sudden and dramatic turn for the worse which will increase my chances for a heart but decrease my odds for survival or I've just got a damn cold that once shaken, will find me again relatively stable and back on the Godforsaken wait list. . . . I had this horrible fear of a perfect donor match turning up and my not being able to accept it for ancillary reasons. . . .

This past weekend my spirits careened about without direction. The anxiety was corrosive and I spent too much time in anger and disbelief. For the most part there was a numbness, a sense of not caring, of idle refuge. Even in the midst of pure concern for Helen, my children and grandchildren and how this sickness may alter their future, my reigning thoughts became selfish; that this thing has happened, ultimately just to me. I alone am the foremost victim and quite frankly, I can endure that. Perhaps I'm much more of a fatalist than I ever realized. A side of me is without faith in reason or in order. Life is simply experience and for reasons not readily discerned, we attempt to go on. That in the living through this strange misfortune that has befallen me other life continues, seems bizarre. These thoughts are so selfish and so unlike what I believe myself to be, it seems strange they are trickling out of my mind. I consider myself a devout Roman Catholic but these words would seem to deny that.

And yet, for the moment, this is the way I am, floating and remote (and a little drugged up, sick and tired; so very tired). Of course, a great deal of the time I spend wondering why these things have happened at all, particularly to me. I find that at some point along the way the ability to assay ceases. My speculation seems to lead to a dark and frightening periphery, the edge of a vortex of paranoia and rage from which (fortunately) I can still quickly withdraw. I know that on some levels I cannot take much more and I simply don't. I push it aside. I worry instead about when it will be over, and what the result will be. I want, with a desperation whose size cannot be encompassed by metaphor, I want all of this never to have taken place; I want things to be as they were before I let my life be ransacked by heart disease and all that followed.

Most of all I need refreshment, a rebirth into the life I have already spent a great deal of myself in carving. To wait eight months for a heart transplant would try the soul of the strongest man. I wonder what a woman feels waiting for the birth of a child. Pain, agony, fear and yet it must be far outweighed by the ultimate outcome, the pure joy of new life. I want that. I want it desperately, but I want it not at the sacrifice of the life of another. And yet that's what I pray for—it's a fool's prayer, a prayer of someone too young to die and too old to weep.

I want no more weekends like the one just past. I'm rarely morose. I see humor in virtually every human transaction. Let's have no more of these black thoughts. I have places to go and things to do and love to share in a life that is bereft of sadness. That's where I belong. Not in the doldrums of despair, but on a pinnacle of a hill watching the rising of the sun on a life that has many years yet to meet. [April 3–May 16]

It was at this time that George began to think he was really close to getting his new heart. He was twice phoned by the transplant coordinator to alert him to be available, but each time it proved to be a false alarm.

The reaction on a patient who has been waiting nine months for these calls is amusing in a jaded sense. First you throw up, then you try to sleep (absurd). This situation probably keyed my current anxieties, but believe me; returning to my former state of limbo may well be impossible. . . . If this be the last note of this series, so be it. I pray the next one will be from a joyfully recovering patient.

All this time, George's health was continuing to deteriorate. The cold had left him with a shortness of breath even more marked than before. Of course, his worsening condition had put him higher on the transplant list, but that was small comfort to a man who had now begun to grapple with the imminence of possible death.

[M]y mental outlook is awful. I'm preoccupied with my symptoms (panting, short-termed exhaustion, minor leg pain). . . . I feel weak, threatened and helpless—and this from a man who has spent his entire life with an abundance of pride in his physical and mental prowess. If I saw my symptoms in another person, I would be intolerant. I deplore weakness in others—to see it in myself is a strange weight to bear.

In that same "Musings," he wrote for the first time of another feeling to which he was unaccustomed: "a number of things perhaps summed up in a single word—fear, an emotion so alien to me that I question not how, but whether I am capable of effectively coping with it." He was losing confidence in his ability to go on and questioning whether "a psychiatrist might bolster my flagging spirits," because "I'm on the rim of being out of control which is a new and completely unpleasant sensation." [May 17–June 20]

By then, early June, George's condition was worsening so rapidly that he needed to be hospitalized for five weeks. He was carrying at least twenty-five pounds of excess fluid and was short of breath most of the time, even at rest. His name was now at the top of the waiting list. One morning during the first week of June, a member of the transplant team unexpectedly came to his room to tell him that a donor heart meeting his specifications had been identified and that preparations for the operation were under way.

Things began to move very swiftly. New tests were taken (blood samples), all food and drink ceased, the usual medications did not take place and lots of fresh faces appeared to prod and poke. New X-rays were taken, IV's were attached, various people came in and told me various things (little of which was retained since the level of excitement, personally as well as with the nurses attending me, was so high as to make everything a blur). I called my family and a few close friends with whatever information I could glean. The atmosphere around me was electric and my blood pressure rose to almost normal. In short, it was tightly controlled chaos and a very happy environment. I was ecstatic. Thousands of prayers were being answered and my dear wife was racing back to the hospital (she was in Maryland at our beach house) to join me.

One of the people George called was me. I, too, was at a beach house, this one on Fire Island, off the shore of Long Island. I caught the next ferry back to the mainland and drove as fast as seemed reasonable to reach my friend's side. When I got there, all was quiet and strangely serene around George's room.

Around noon (the operation was scheduled for late afternoon) the euphoria came to a sudden halt. A final tissue test match done in Boston that morning indicated a high probability of rejection. The local decision was easy. It was a no-go. All preparations ceased and immediately everything returned to normal. The atmosphere of disappointment was palpable, not only with me, but with the dozens of people involved in the pre-operation procedures. It was a difficult scene, frustration in its worst form. . . . All in all, it was a fascinating experience—one I'd rather not repeat but nonetheless an adventure that further convinced me that a solution to my specific problem was at hand. It was (is) only a matter of time.

Discharge from the hospital took place a few weeks later, and a somewhat improved George Leyden went home to resume the wait. His excess fluid was gone, his breathing was easier, and the flurry of activity had renewed some of his badly damaged optimism. On August 9, he wrote me from home:

I rarely think about my situation except when asked. To do so would only sadden me, and I refuse to let that occur. To counteract the dreadful thoughts that lay hidden in the recesses of my mind, I focus on any number of other things. . . . There is no way I can let myself be dominated by fear, but I can never lapse into a feeling of security despite the strength gathered from my religion and my periodic sense of well being. A sense of fatalism would be of great help, but that's not part of my makeup. I've always believed the *Invictus* line about being "master of my fate; captain of my soul" has a degree of merit. The statistical helplessness of the situation may occasionally drive me batty, but up to the present I've at least warded off enough of the demons to give the appearance of sanity (I think).

That was to be George's last letter. He began to feel some mild chest pain on the following morning, which increased with each passing day, as did his shortness of breath when in any position other than fully upright. On August 15, he was readmitted to the Yale–New Haven Hospital and vigorous attempts were made to treat the worsening heart failure. Only partially successful, these efforts were complicated by the development of serious disturbances of cardiac rhythm. At 6:50 P.M. on Friday, August 26, George's heart arrested during an attempt to pass a Swan-Ganz catheter to monitor fluid status. He was resuscitated and put on a respirator, but another episode occurred four hours later, after which it was obvious that he had sustained major brain damage. He began having seizures at about 4:00 A.M. and his great heart finally came to a stop two hours later.

Almost thirty years have passed since the Saturday morning when I stood alongside George Leyden's body in a small glass-walled cubicle of Yale–New Haven's cardiac intensive care unit, the curtain pulled so that we could be alone for one last time. I muttered at him under my breath, scarcely able to control my anger that he had left me. Sorrow, rage, frustration at losing this extraordinary friend and everything that his new life would bring him—even now, with so long to look back on it, I have no idea why I found the emotions so uncontrollable or why so much of the anger was directed at the dead body of the man whose life had meant so much to me. Later, I tried not to take out my feelings on the young attending physician in charge of the unit, but I could speak to him only through gritted teeth, as though he and only he were the cause of the spiraling of events that had taken George from me. To this day, I see that doctor from time to time, now middle-aged and prosperous, and I cannot look into his eyes without the choking resentment rising in my throat, though I know it has no justification.

Much later, I did write that article for *The New Yorker*, but I chose to meet its subject when he was already on the operating table and anesthetized. I told myself that I had made the decision to proceed in that way because I could not bear the possibility of making a friend again, and then losing him. But I had long known that, for me, there would never be another George Leyden, and no quality of sorrow at all like what I had felt when he died. The man about whom I eventually wrote following his successful surgery told me that in order to fulfill what was necessary to endure the roller coaster of awaiting his transplant and then persevere through the ordeal of its aftermath, he had had to rise to "a step above—a step above what I usually am—so I could do what I had to do." When his name was placed on the waiting list, George Leyden was already a step above this man, a step above me, and a step above the vast majority of the rest of us.

ACKNOWLEDGMENTS

The spring issue of 1998 began a new era in the sixty-six-year history of *The American Scholar*, with the appointment of Anne Fadiman as editor. Those of us privileged to become members of the editorial board at that time became a kind of fellowship of letters, a team of already-seasoned writers who genuinely enjoyed one another's work—and one another's company at our semiannual meetings and elsewhere—ever more as the quarterly issues came forth one after the other. For a surgeon-turned-author like me, those six years were a period of inspiration.

To be numbered among such talented men and women would have been gift enough, but the ultimate reward was the skilled and sensitive touch of our editor, Anne Fadiman. Those many readers familiar with Anne's writing need no reminder of the luminous contributions she has made to the art of the written word, both in her essays and in her books. But those of us who have been edited by her have had the added advantage of her gentle tact, her understanding ear and eye, and her keen intelligence. I learned a great deal about the essay form in those years, and I found a muse who knew how to maximize the creativity of a group of independent-minded people, every one of whom had already achieved some eminence. Except for the last, each of the chapters in this book is a slight modification of one of the sequence of essays I wrote for Anne Fadiman during the time I was a contributing editor to *The American Scholar* between 1998 and 2004.

None of *The Scholar*'s success could have been achieved without the constant care and meticulous oversight of its longtime managing editor, Jean Stipikevic. Jean's touch was everywhere, and we contributors were thankful that every comma and every deadline was being watched over by her, as they were by Sandra Costich, our associate editor. For a man like me—brought up in a matriarchal family—to be in the hands of such a triumvirate of capable women seemed the most natural thing in the world.

I am grateful also to Dr. Lawrence Cohen, not only for having introduced me to George Leyden, but for being such a good friend for these many years. George could not have had a more devoted or competent physician—and neither could the legions of men and women who have been Larry Cohen's patients.

Helen Leyden, "the most beautiful girl I had ever seen," was the deep vein of strength in George's life, and was—along with his own inherent inner resilience—the underlying reason, I am convinced, that he was able to persevere in spite of one setback after another. I don't know how much confidence she had in the doctors, the hospital, or in the contemporary state of the art of medicine, but Helen's invincible faith in her husband's human spirit never lessened, and he knew it. "There is a land of the living and a land of the dead," wrote my Hamden neighbor Thornton Wilder, "and the bridge is love."

INDEX

abdominal surgery, 45, 46
abortion, 5
academic medicine, 20–27, 28–34
acupuncture, 42–49
    endorphins, 51, 52, 54, 58
    gate theory, 51, 52
    surgical, 42–49, 50–58
    thyroid surgery under, 45, 46–49,
        50, 52–53
    Western science on, 51–52
Adams, Francis, 3
aerobic exercise, 38
Aesculapius, 144
Agency for Healthcare Research and
    Quality, xvii
aging, 63–64, 143
    "compression of morbidity," 64
    loss of muscle strength and, 37,
        38
Agnew, Hayes, 156
alcohol, 42
American Association for the History
    of Medicine, 158
American College of Physicians,
    100
American College of Sports Medicine,
    38
American College of Surgeons, 32,
    33
    Bulletin, 32
American Medical Association, 23–24,
    151
    Bureau of Investigation, 137

Council on Medical Education, 23
anaerobic exercise, 38, 41
anatomy, 62, 92–93, 110–111, 112
    Gray's Anatomy, 113–15
    murder, 95–97
    procurement of cadavers, 91–98
Anatomy Act (1832), 97
Anderson, W. French, 61
anesthesia, 42–43, 127, 128, 129
    acupuncture, 42–49, 50–58
    cocaine as, 163
    history of, 42–43
anesthesiology, 42–43, 126, 127
Angell, James Rowland, 21
anger, 69, 70
anima, 73
antibiotics, 17, 101, 102, 105
apprenticeship system, 22
Aristotle, 70
Armstrong, P. M., 91
art, 148–56
    The Gross Clinic, 149–56
arteriosclerosis, 63, 133
arthritis, 63
assisted suicide, 5
Association of American Medical
    Colleges, 32, 33
    "Physicians for the 21st Century"
        (study), 32
Atlas, Charles, 136
Australia, 97
autointoxication, 135–39
autonomy, 144–45, 146

back pain, low, 57
Bacon, Francis, *Novum organum*, 112
bacteria, 134–35
bacteriology, xiv, 28
battlefield injuries, 63
Beijing, 42, 49
Bernard, Claude, 8
    *Introduction to Experimental
        Medicine*, 8–9
bile, 69
    black, 68, 69–70, 112, 134
    yellow, 68, 69, 112, 134
bioethics, 16–17
biology, 28, 29, 111
biometrics, 63
biopsies, 61
Bizzozero, Joe, 106–107
black bile, 68, 69–70, 112, 134
blistering, 68
blood, 68
    circulation of, 112
    as humor, 68, 69, 70–71, 112
    transfusion, 102
Bologna, 22, 161
bone density, 35, 38
books, medical, 108–115
*Boston Medical and Surgical Journal,
    The*, 113, 114
Boston Medical Library, 115
Bouchard, Charles, 135
    Lectures in Autointoxication, 135
bowel regularity, 132–39
brain, 35, 55, 63, 69, 103, 104
    electroshock therapy, 123–31
    endorphins, 51, 54
    surgery, 46, 56
    tumors, 46
breast cancer, xvi, 7–8
Brevital, 127
Brown University, xvi
*Bulletin of the Institute for the History of
    Medicine*, 3, 4
Burke, William, 96–97
burke (term), 96
Bush, George W., 17

Cabanis, Pierre, 120, 121
cadavers, procurement of, 91–98
Calcar, Jan Stephan van, 111
California Institute of Technology,
    157
cancer, 7, 133
    breast, xvi, 7–8
    diagnosis of, 7–8
    liver, 52
    lymphatic, 104
    new technologies and, 62
    prostate, 73
    surgery, 62, 102
Cao Xiaoding, 53–55
Capp, Al, "Li'l Abner," 75
carbolic acid antisepsis, 151, 155
cardiac episodes in public places,
    75–82
cardiac transplantation, 165–85
cardiomyopathy, 168, 169, 171
cardiopulmonary resuscitation, 77
cardiovascular disease, 37, 62
cardiovascular exercise, 40
Carlyle, Thomas, 160
Carnegie Foundation for the
    Advancement of Teaching, 24, 28
Cartesian dualism, 103
Cascade, 136–37
case histories, 88–89
Catholicism, 92–93, 180
caudate nucleus, 54
causation of disease, 29
cells, rejuvenated, 14
Celsus, xix
    De medicina, xix
Changsha, 42, 44, 45–49
chemistry, 29
chest surgery, 45, 46, 49
chi, 47, 49, 50, 58
childbed fever, 161–62
China, 42–49, 50–58
    acupuncture anesthesia in, 42–49,
        50–58
    Cultural Revolution, 52
    medicine, 42–49, 50–58

chiropractic, 99
chloroform, 42
cholesterol, 41
chronic low back pain, 57
cigarettes, 146
clinical studies, xvii, 25
Clinton, Bill, 16
cloning, 12–19
    ethics and, 16–17
    human, 13, 16
    mouse, 12–13
Clow, Roderick, 91–98
cocaine, as anesthesia, 163
Coffin, William Sloane, 107
Cohen, Lawrence, 167, 168, 171, 179
Columbia-Presbyterian Medical
    Center, 81
Columbia University, 22
compliance, patient, 140–47
"compression of morbidity," 64
confidentiality, 88–89
congenital diseases, 62, 63
consciousness, 63
constipation, 132–39
convulsions, 124
Cooper, Sir Astley, 94, 97
Copernicus, *De revolutionibus orbium
    coelestium*, 159
Cos, 4
cosmetic surgery, 18
Cramp, Arthur J., 137
Crouch, 92
CT scans, 38, 62
cupping, 68
cure of disease, 7, 29, 32

Daumier, Honoré, 149
death, 32, 37, 174
    anatomy murder, 95–97
    cardiac arrest, 75–79, 184
    grave robbing, 91–98
    grief after 9/11, 116–22
    group avoidance and, 75–79
    holiday-related, 103
degrees, medical, 22–27

Demerol, 47
democracy, 120, 121
depression, 70
    electroshock therapy for, 123–31
diabetes, 102, 138
diagnosis, xv, xvi, 7–8, 10, 113
    of cancer, 7–8
    early, 7–8, 17
*Diagnostic and Statistical Manual of the
    American Psychiatric Association,*
    72
diagnostic imaging, 61–62
diet, 17, 40
digestion, 104, 138
disease, xv, 7, 35, 59, 120
    causation of, 29
    cure of, 7, 29, 32
    First Aphorism and, 3–11
    germ theory of, 59, 134–35, 138,
        151–56, 161–62
    humors theory, 68–71, 92, 112–13,
        134
    molecular origins of, 60–62
    new technologies and, 59–66
    prevention of, 17, 29
    spread of, 29
dissection, human, 92–93
    procurement of cadavers for, 91–98
DNA, 14, 64, 102, 109
    discovery of, 159
Docherty, Margaret, 96
doctor-patient relationship, 9–10, 101
Dolly (sheep), 13
dopamine, 126
droperidol, 47
drugs, 18
Dürer, Albrecht, 149
Dyson, Freeman, 157

Eakins, Thomas, 149–56
    The Agnew Clinic, 149, 156
    The Gross Clinic, 149–56
Eclectic Institute, 137
economy, 21
Edinburgh, 93, 96–97

education, medical, xiii, xiv, 20–27, 28–34
    American system of, 20–26, 30
    European model, 22, 23, 24
    Flexner Report, 24–25, 28–31
    humanities and, 32–34
    Johns Hopkins model, 24
    procurement of cadavers for, 91–98
Egyptians, 133–34
elderly, 36
    exercise and, 36, 37, 38–41
electrocardiograms, 61
electroconvulsive therapy (ECT), 123–31
electroencephalogram, 127
electrogenicity, 36
Eliot, T. S., 19
emetics, 68
emotions, 67–68, 84–85, 89
    grief after 9/11, 116–22
    theory of humors, 68–71
Empedocles, 69
empyema, 105–106
endocrine system, 104
end-of-life care, 32
endorphins, acupuncture-induced, 51, 52, 54, 58
enemas, 68, 133, 134
Epidemics, 121
epidemiology, 25
epilepsy, 34, 124, 138
Epstein, Lynn C., xvi
ether, 42
ethics, 5, 16–19, 32, 89
Europe, 43, 54, 111, 149, 151
    medical education in, 22, 23, 24, 92
evidence-based medicine, xvii
exercise, 35–41
    aerobic, 38
    life expectancy and, 36–37
    weight training, 37, 38–41
experience, 8–9

Fadiman, Anne, The Spirit Catches You and You Fall Down, 34

faith, 63
fast food, 146
Fildes, Luke, 149
First Aphorism (Hippocrates), xiv–xv, 3–11, 142, 143, 145–46
Flexner, Abraham, 24–25, 28–31, 32, 33
Flexner Report, 24–25, 28–31
foolishness, 18
France, 22, 134
free association, 86
Freud, Sigmund, 10
functional magnetic resonance imaging (fMRI), 61
funding, federal, 25–26

Galen, 70, 99, 103, 105, 109–110, 111, 112, 160–61
gallstones, 133
gastric ulcer, 138
gate theory, 51, 52
gene therapy, 60–61, 62
genetics, 13, 18, 25, 33, 60–61, 64
genome, 64
Genuine Works of Hippocrates, The, 3
Germany, 21
    medical education in, 23, 24
germ theory, 59, 134–35, 138, 151–56, 161–62
    The Gross Clinic and, 151–56
"Gesundheit," 74
Gibbon, Edward, The History of the Decline and Fall of the Roman Empire, 108
globus hystericus, 71
Goya, Francisco, 149
grave robbing, 91–98
Gray, Henry, 113–14
    Gray's Anatomy, 113–15
Great Books, 108, 115
Great Britain, 22, 98, 151
    bowel obsessions, 132, 136–39
    medical education in, 22, 92, 93, 98
    provision of instructional cadavers, 93–98

Greeks, 4, 6, 12, 68, 73, 74, 99, 103, 121, 142, 144, 145, 148, 160
  theory of humors, 68–71, 112, 134
Greenfield, Marsha, 57
grief, 116–17
  after 9/11, 116–22
Gross, Samuel David, 151–56
Gross, Samuel W., 156
Gross Clinic, The (Eakins), 149–56
group avoidance, and illness, 75–79
Guy's Hospital, London, xiii, 97, 137

Hall, A. Wilford, 136
Halsted, William, 140, 141, 163
Halstedian technique, 163
Hare, William, 96–97
Harvard University, 22, 36, 114
Harvey, William, 111–12, 115, 159
  Exercitatio anatomica de motu cordis et sanguinis in animalibus, 111–12
Hastings Institute, xviii
Hawthorne, Nathaniel, 85, 114
healing, 34, 101–102, 104–105
heart, 67, 69
  surgery, 49
  transplant, 165–85
heart disease, 37, 62, 162
  cardiac episodes in public places, 75–82
  heart transplants, 165–85
high colonics, 68
Hillel, 6
Hippocrates, xiv, xix, 3–11, 12, 99, 103, 121, 142–45, 149
  The Aphorisms, 3–11, 12
  background of, 4
  death of, 7
  First Aphorism, xiv–xv, 3–11, 142, 143, 145–46
  writings and philosophy, 3–11, 12, 121, 142–45
Hippocratic Oath, 5
historians, medical, 157–64
HIV triple-drug therapy, 142
Holbein the Younger, Hans, 149

holiday-related deaths, 103
Holmes, Oliver Wendell, 35, 114–15
homeopathy, xiv, 99
hormones, 41, 67
hospitals, 17, 144
  medical schools affiliated with, 29–30
  medical teaching in, 22, 23
Hou Lihui, 46–49
Houston, W. R., 100–101
human condition, 84, 90
humanism, xix, 21, 32–34
humanities, 32–34
human potential movement, 18
humors, 68–71, 92, 112–13, 134
  black bile, 68, 69–70, 113, 134
  blood, 68, 69, 70–71, 113
  phlegm, 68, 69, 113
  yellow bile, 68, 69, 113, 134
Hunan Medical University, 42, 45, 46, 56
Hunter, John, 62
Hurst, Sir Arthur, 139
Huxley, Aldous, 58, 85
hygiene, 17, 145
hypnosis, 42
"hysteria," theory of, 71–72

immune system, 104
immunization, 17, 145
infectious diseases, xvi
Institute of Human Relations, 20–21, 26–27, 29
insulin, 102
internal medicine, 25, 26
International Medical Congress, 151, 154
International Physicians for the Prevention of Nuclear War, xvii, 146
intestine, 46
in vitro fertilization, 13
Islam, 121
Israel, 103
Italy, 22, 124–25

Jefferson Medical College, 151, 152, 154, 156
Johns Hopkins Hospital, 140
Johns Hopkins Medical School, xiv, 24, 163
Johns Hopkins University, xiv, 3, 20
Journal of Sports Sciences, 37
Journal of the American Medical Association, The, 137
Journal of the History of Medicine and Allied Sciences, 158
journals, medical, 85, 89, 108, 109, 113, 114
judgment, 9–11
junk food, 146
Juvenal, 35

Keats, John, xiii, xiv, xix
    Endymion, xiii
Kellogg, John Harvey, 135
King's College, 22
King's College Hospital, London, 97
Knox, Robert, 96
Kocher clamp, 48

Laënnec, René-Théophile-Hyacinthe, xiv, 162–63
Lancet, The, 95, 97, 109, 113
Landers, Ann, 36
Lane, William Arbuthnot, 137–39
language, 67–74
    "hysteria," 71–72
    medical writing and, 88–90
    theory of humors, 68–71
laser surgery, 62
Lavoisier, Antoine, 159
"Law" (essay), 12, 17
laxatives, 134
Lehrfreiheit und Lernfreiheit, 23
Leonardo da Vinci, 93
Leyden, George, 165–85
Liao, Sung, 56–58
life, laboratory creation of, 64

life expectancy, 6–7, 17, 63–64, 120
    cloning and, 13–14
    exercise and, 36–37
Lister, Joseph, 134, 151, 152, 153, 155, 156, 162
Liston, Robert, 92
literature, 31, 32
liver, 67, 69, 71, 111
    cancer, 52
    terminology, 71
Locke, John, 35
    Some Thoughts Concerning Education, 35
London, 56, 92, 93, 97
    grave robbing, 93–94
Longfellow, Henry Wadsworth, 60, 172
    "The Ladder of Saint Augustine," 66
Lonsdale, Henry, 94
low back pain, 57
lungs, 46
lymphoma, 104

Macfadden, Bernarr, 136
mammography, 8
Mann, Felix, 56–57, 58
Mao Zedong, 43, 46, 55
Marshall Plan, 121
Massachusetts General Hospital, 56
media, 14, 144
medical history, 157–64
medical schools, xiv, 6, 20–27, 28–34
    American system of, 22–26, 30
    curriculum, 32–34
    European model, 22, 23, 24
    Flexner Report, 24–25, 28–31
    humanities and, 32–34
    Johns Hopkins model, 24
    procurement of cadavers, 91–98
medicine, 16
    academic, 20–27, 28–34
    artist and, 148–56
    books, 108–115
    bowel regularity, 132–39

Chinese, 42–49, 50–58
dehumanization of, 27
evidence-based, xvii
First Aphorism and, 3–11
heart transplantation, 165–85
historians of, 157–64
language, 67–74
mind/body connection and, 99–107
new technologies, 59–66
nineteenth-century, xiii–xiv, 23, 59, 68, 91–98, 113–15, 134–35, 140, 145, 149–56
patient compliance, 140–47
procurement of cadavers, 91–98
uncertainty of, xv, xvi, xvii, 118
writing, 88–90
melancholy, and spleen, 70
Mesmer, Anton, 99
Metamucil, 132
Metchnikoff, Élie, 135–36
  The Nature of Man, 138
  The Prolongation of Life, 137
Metropolitan Museum of Art, New York, 154
mice, cloning, 12–13
Michelangelo, 93
Middle Ages, 72
Mill, John Stuart, 28
mind/body connection, 63, 99–107
molecular biology, 12–15, 17, 18, 25, 33, 59
Monro, Alexander, 96–97
Montaigne, Michel de, 87
Montpellier, 22
Morgagni, Giovanni, 112–13, 115
  De sedibus et causis morborum per anatomen indagatis, 112–13
mortsafe, 95
mourning, after 9/11, 116–22
MRI, 62
muscle relaxants, 127, 128
muscle strength, 35, 37, 38
  loss of, 37, 38
mustard plasters, 68

narcissism, 18
National Academy of Sciences, 43
National Bioethics Advisory Commission, 16–17
National Institutes of Health (NIH), 25
"A Natural History of Athleticism, Health and Longevity" (article), 37
Nature, 109
nerves, 35–36, 55
  electrogenicity, 36
nervous system, 54–55, 67, 104
neurobiology, 53
neurosurgery, 33
neurotransmitters, 126
New England Journal of Medicine, The, 7, 109, 113
New Haven Register, 103
Newton, Isaac, 157
New York, 75, 132, 154
New Yorker, The, 167, 184
New York Review of Books, The, 157
New York Times, 12, 14, 173
New York University College of Medicine, 56
9/11, grief and reflection after, 116–22
nitrous oxide, 42
noncompliance, patient, 140–47
norepinephrine, 126
nursing, 16

open-heart surgery, 49
Oporinus, Joannes, 111
orchid, 73
orchiectomy, 73
organ transplants, 13, 59, 63
  heart, 165–85
orgasm, doctor-induced, 72
Osler, William, xiv, xv, xviii
osteomyelitis, 153
osteoporosis, 38
outcomes research, xvii

pain control, with acupuncture, 42–49, 50–58
Pancoast, Joseph, 152
Paracelsus, 124
Paré, Ambroise, 73
Paris, xiv, 22, 152, 161
  hospitals, 23
Pascal, Blaise, *Pensées*, 65
Pasteur, Louis, 134, 135, 151, 153, 159
pathology, 28
pediatrics, 25
Peking Union Medical College, 49, 55
Pennsylvania Academy of the Fine Arts, 152
Pennsylvania Hospital, 151–52
peptic ulcer, xvi
periaqueductal gray matter (PAG), 54, 55
"personal fulfillment" cult, 19
pharmacogenomics, 102
pharmacology, 17
phenobarbital, 47
Philadelphia, 151, 152, 154, 155
Philadelphia Museum of Art, 154
phlegm, as humor, 68, 69, 112
phren, 67–68
phrenology, 68
physicians, 9–10, 146–47
  artists and, 148–56
  cardiac episodes in public places and, 75–82
  derivation of the word, 146–47
  education of, 12, 20–27, 28–34
  experience, 8–9
  First Aphorism and, 3–11
  judgment, 9–11
  mind, body, and, 99–107
  orgasm induced by, 72
  patient compliance with, 140–47
  therapeutic power of physician's goodness, 99–107
physics, 29
physiology, xiv
placebos, 63, 99–101
Plato, *Timaeus*, 71–72

poverty, 120, 145
Precepts, 145
pregnancy, 72
President's Council on Bioethics, 17
prevention of disease, 17, 29
Princeton University, 12
productivity, 36
Project on the Goals of Medicine, xviii
prostate cancer, 73
psyche, 73, 103–104
psychic pneuma, 109
psychoneuroimmunology, 104
psychosomatic symptoms, 72
public health, 145, 146
punch in the jaw, 42
purging, 68, 134

Rand, Benjamin Howard, 152–53
regularity, bowel, 132
religion, 16, 120
Rembrandt van Rijn, 149
Renaissance, 72, 149
research, xiv, 16, 24–26, 65, 109
  funding, 25–26
  new technologies, 61–62, 63
  outcomes, xvii
  stem cell, 17, 63
  university, 24–26, 30
resistance training, 37, 38–41
responsibility, medical, 145–46
Reston, James, 55–56, 58
rete mirabile, 109, 110
Revolutionary War, 22
Reynolds, Joshua, 149
rheumatoid arthritis, 138
Rivera, Diego, 149
Rockefeller Foundation, 55
Romans, 67
Rome, 125
rotator cuff syndrome, 56
Rousseau, Jean Jacques, *Confessions*, 166
Rowlandson, Thomas, 149
Royal College of Surgeons, xiii

St. Andrew's University, 28
St. Thomas's Hospital, London, 56
sanitation, 145
Sargent, John Singer, 149
scatological medicine, 132–39
Science, 37, 109
Scotland, 93
Semmelweis, Ignác, 161–62
September 11 terrorist attacks, grief
    and reflection after, 116–22
serotonin, 126
Serutan, 132
sex, 72–73
    doctor-induced orgasm, 72
    theory of "hysteria" and, 72
Shakespeare, William, *Hamlet,* 167
Shanghai, 42, 52–56
Shanghai Medical University, 52–55
Shaw, George Bernard, *The Doctor's
    Dilemma,* 138
Shelley, Percy Bysshe, 20, 86
Shepherd of the Anus, 133–34
Sixtus IV, Pope, 92
snake, 105
sneeze, 73–74
socioeconomic conditions, and health,
    21, 145–46
soul, 73
    loss of, 73, 74
spleen, 67, 70
    black bile and, 70
    melancholy and, 71
Sprague, Ruth, 91–92, 98
spread of disease, 29
staphylococcus, 105
State University of New York,
    56–57
statistics, 9, 25
steam room, 68
stem cell research, 17, 63
steroids, 58
stethoscope, invention of, 113,
    162–63
stomach, 67
suffocation, 96

surgery, 17, 25, 26, 59, 83
    acupuncture anesthesia for, 42–49,
        50–58
    brain, 46, 56
    cancer, 62, 102
    early forms of pain relief, 42–43
    exploratory, 61
    future of, 62
    heart, 49
    medical history and, 161–64
    new technologies and, 62–63
    polarity between writing and,
        83–84
    procurement of cadavers and,
        91–98
    thyroid, 45, 46–49
survivors' guilt, 116
sweating, 68
Sydenham Society of London, 3

Talmud, 6
Tang Zhaoyou, 52–53
technology, 16, 59–66, 148
    cloning, 12–19
    new, 59–66
telomerase, 14
telomere, 14
Teniers, David, 149
testicles, 73
testosterone, 41
therapy, xv, xvi, 7, 10, 113
    electroconvulsive, 123–31
    gene, 60–61, 62
    new technologies, 59–66
Thomson, Mowbray, 92
thyroid disease, 138
thyroid surgery, under acupuncture,
    45, 46–49, 50, 52–53
time, 6–7
tissue transplants, 13
Titian, 111
transplantation of organs, 13, 59, 63
    heart, 165–85
trauma, 62–63
tuberculosis, 133

Tufts University, 37
Tyrell, Charles, 136–37
   The Royal Road to Health, 136–37

ulcer:
   gastric, 138
   peptic, xvi
uncertainty, medical, xv, xvi, xvii,
   118
unconscious, 103
   writing and, 85–87
U.S. Centennial Exposition (1876,
   Philadelphia), 151
university-affiliated medical schools,
   20–27, 28–34
University College, London, 92
university medical centers, 30–34
University of Chicago, 7
University of Copenhagen, 100
University of Edinburgh, 22, 96, 97,
   151
University of Minnesota, 158
University of Padua, 110, 161
University of Pennsylvania, 22, 37,
   156
University of Rochester, 104
uterus, 71–73
   theory of "hysteria" and, 71–72

Valium, 53
Venice, 111
Vesalius, Andreas, 110, 112, 115, 161
   De human corporis fabrica, 92,
   110–11, 112, 161
vibrator, 72
Virchow, Rudolf, 21–22, 29, 33, 120,
   121

vital pneuma, 109
Voltaire, 8

war injuries, 63
Watson and Crick, 159
wehuduw, 133
weight training, 37, 38–41
Whitman, Walt, 156
Williams, William Carlos, xix
Wilson, Leonard, 158–59
Winternitz, Milton, 20–22, 26–27, 29,
   32–33
Wordsworth, William, 85
World War II, 101
writing, 83–90
   by heart transplant candidate,
   165–85
   medical, 88–90, 108–115, 157–58
   polarity between surgery and,
   83–84
   unconscious and, 85–87
Wyeth, Andrew, 149

X-rays, 61
Xu Letian, 49
Xu Qiming, 47

Yale-China Association, 42
Yale-New Haven Hospital, 76, 105,
   167, 168, 169, 184
Yale School of Epidemiology and
   Public Health, 57
Yale School of Medicine, 20–22,
   26–27, 29, 42
Yale University, 20–21, 29, 107
Yan Zhangshou, 45–49, 50, 51–52, 58
yellow bile, 68, 69, 112, 134

ABOUT THE TYPE

This book was set in Bell, a typeface which was
introduced by John Bell in England in 1788. The typeface
was cut for Bell's foundry by the notable British punchcutter
Richard Austin. Bell had a resurgence in 1931, when it was
recut by the English Monotype Company and brought to
America in 1932, where it was cut by the Lanston
Monotype Machine Company of Philadelphia.